My First Yoga Book

Written by
Ananya Singh
Khushboo Singh

Om Books International

First Published in 2025 by

Om Books International

Corporate & Editorial Office
A-12, Sector 64, Noida 201 301
Uttar Pradesh, India
Phone: +91 120 477 4100
Email: editorial@ombooks.com
Website: www.ombooksinternational.com

Sales Office
107, Ansari Road, Darya Ganj
New Delhi 110 002, India
Phone: +91 11 4000 9000
Email: sales@ombooks.com

ISBN: 978-93-6395-780-0

Printed in India

10 9 8 7 6 5 4 3 2 1

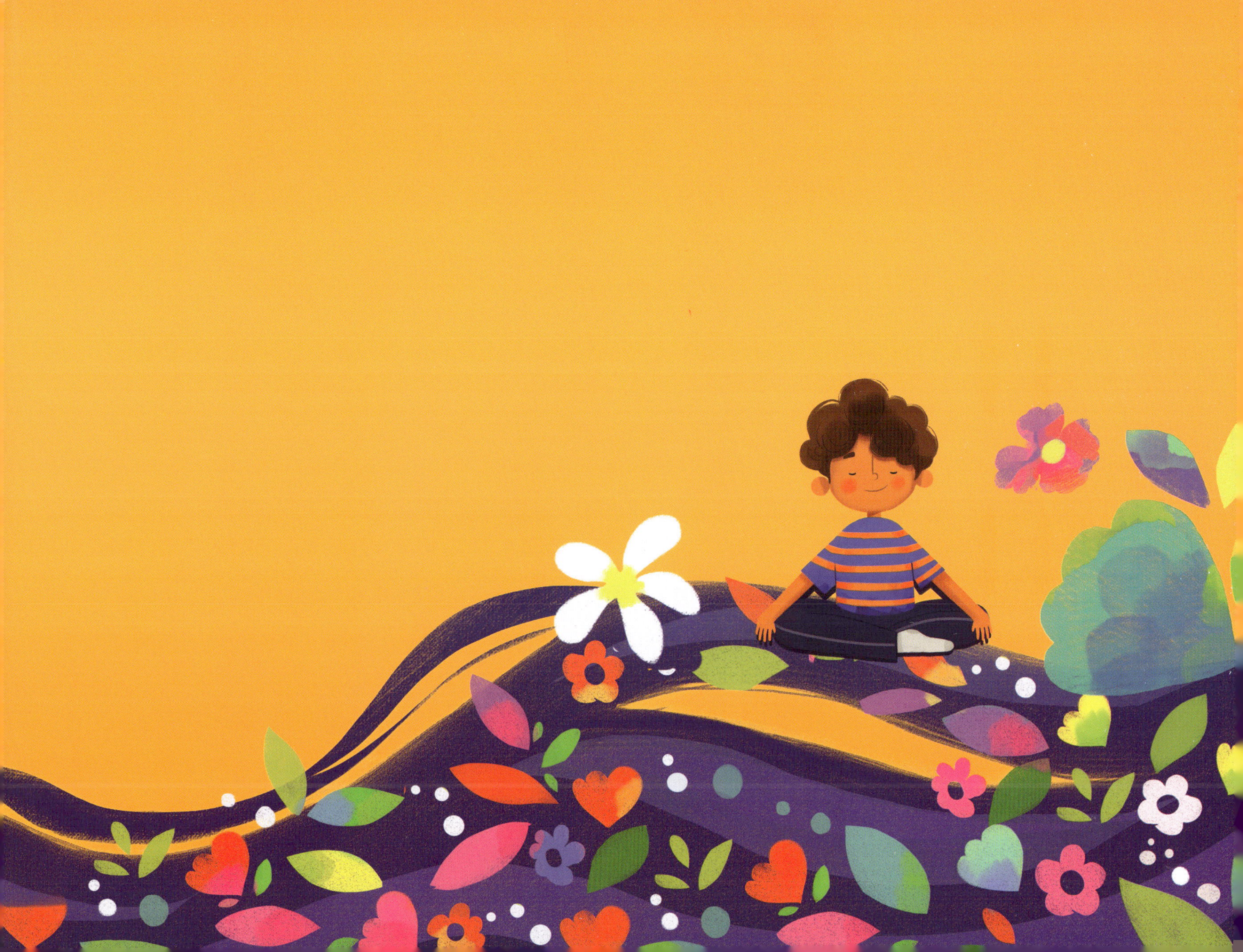

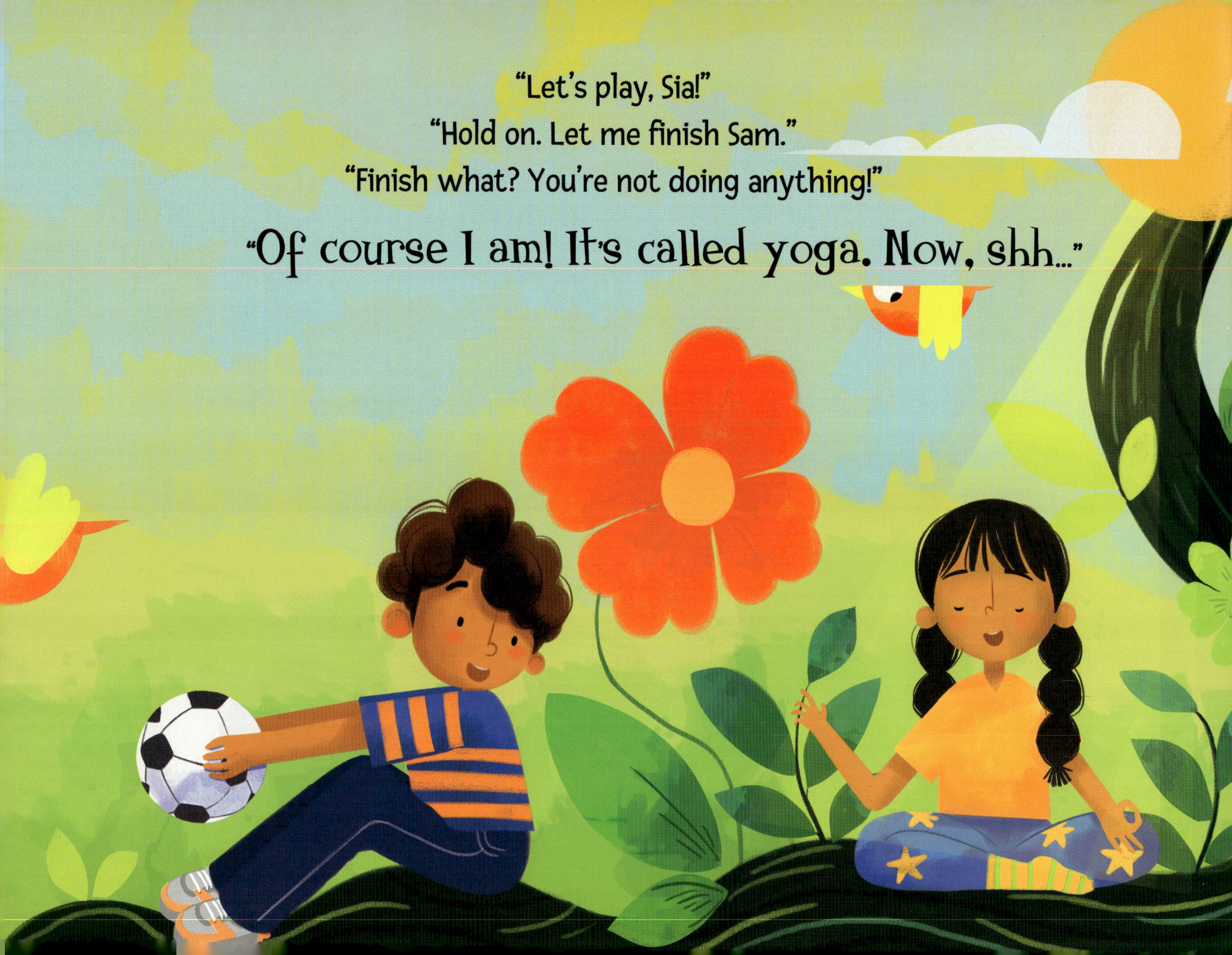

"Let's play, Sia!"
"Hold on. Let me finish Sam."
"Finish what? You're not doing anything!"
"Of course I am! It's called yoga. Now, shh..."

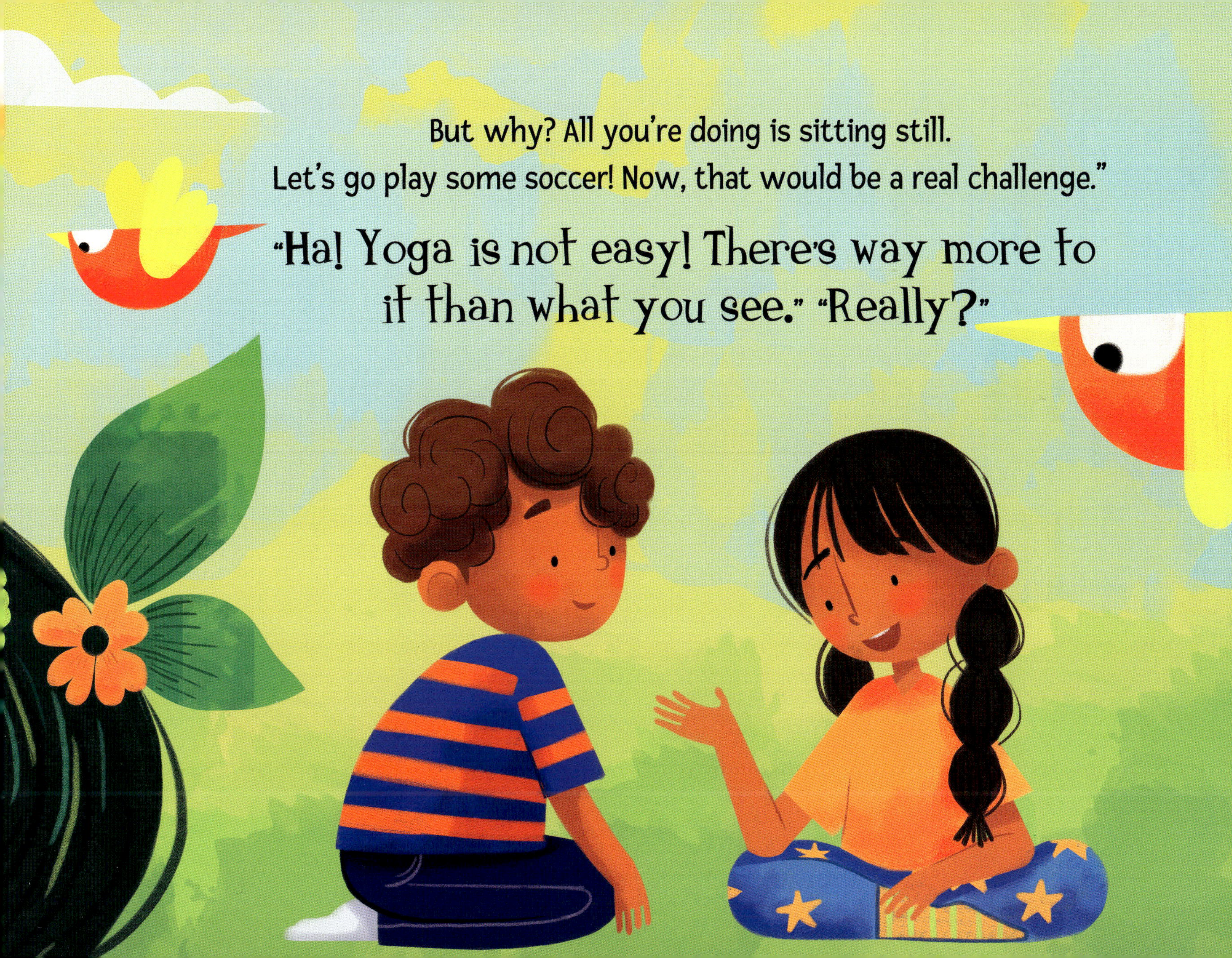

But why? All you're doing is sitting still.
Let's go play some soccer! Now, that would be a real challenge."
"Ha! Yoga is not easy! There's way more to it than what you see." "Really?"

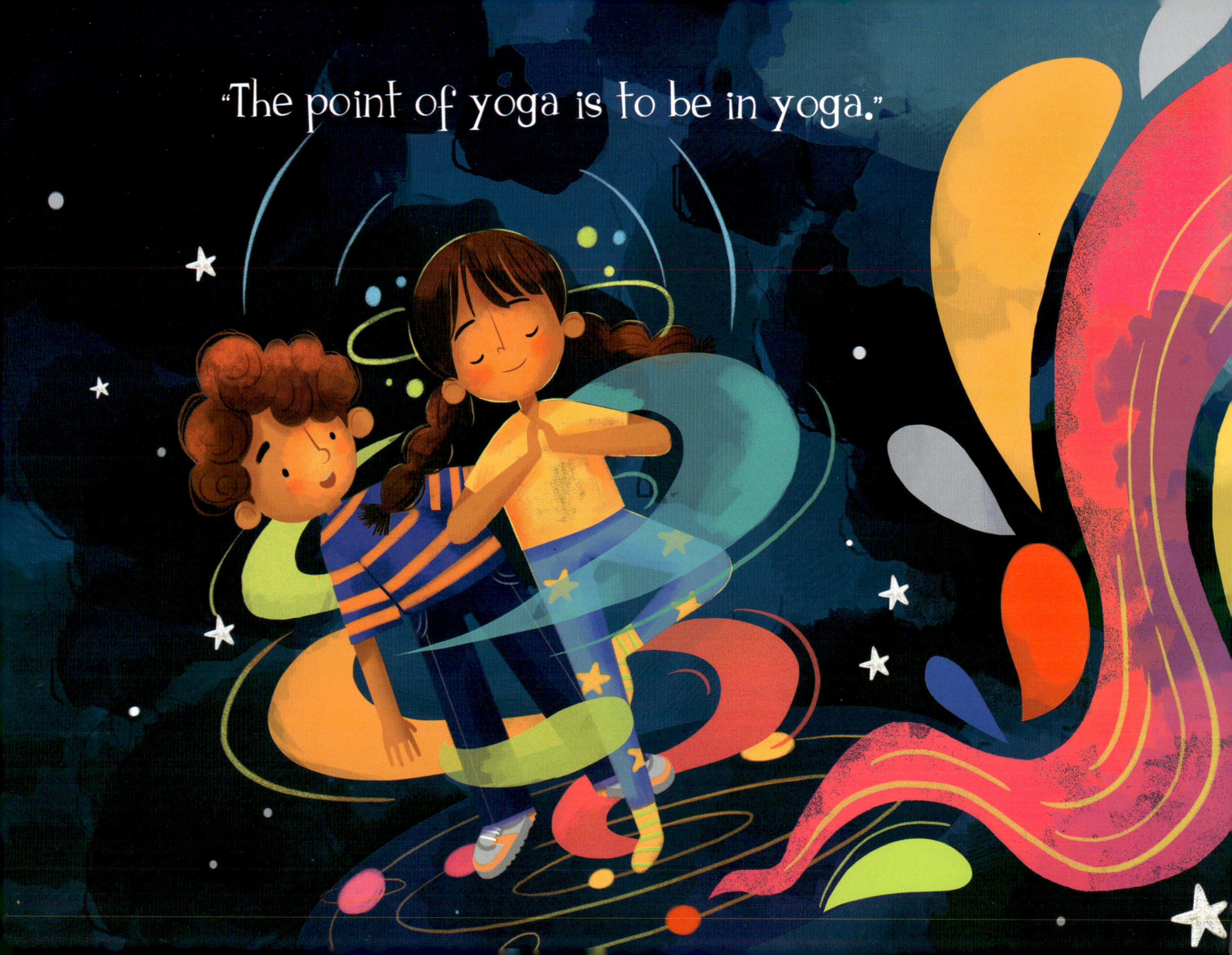
"The point of yoga is to be in yoga."

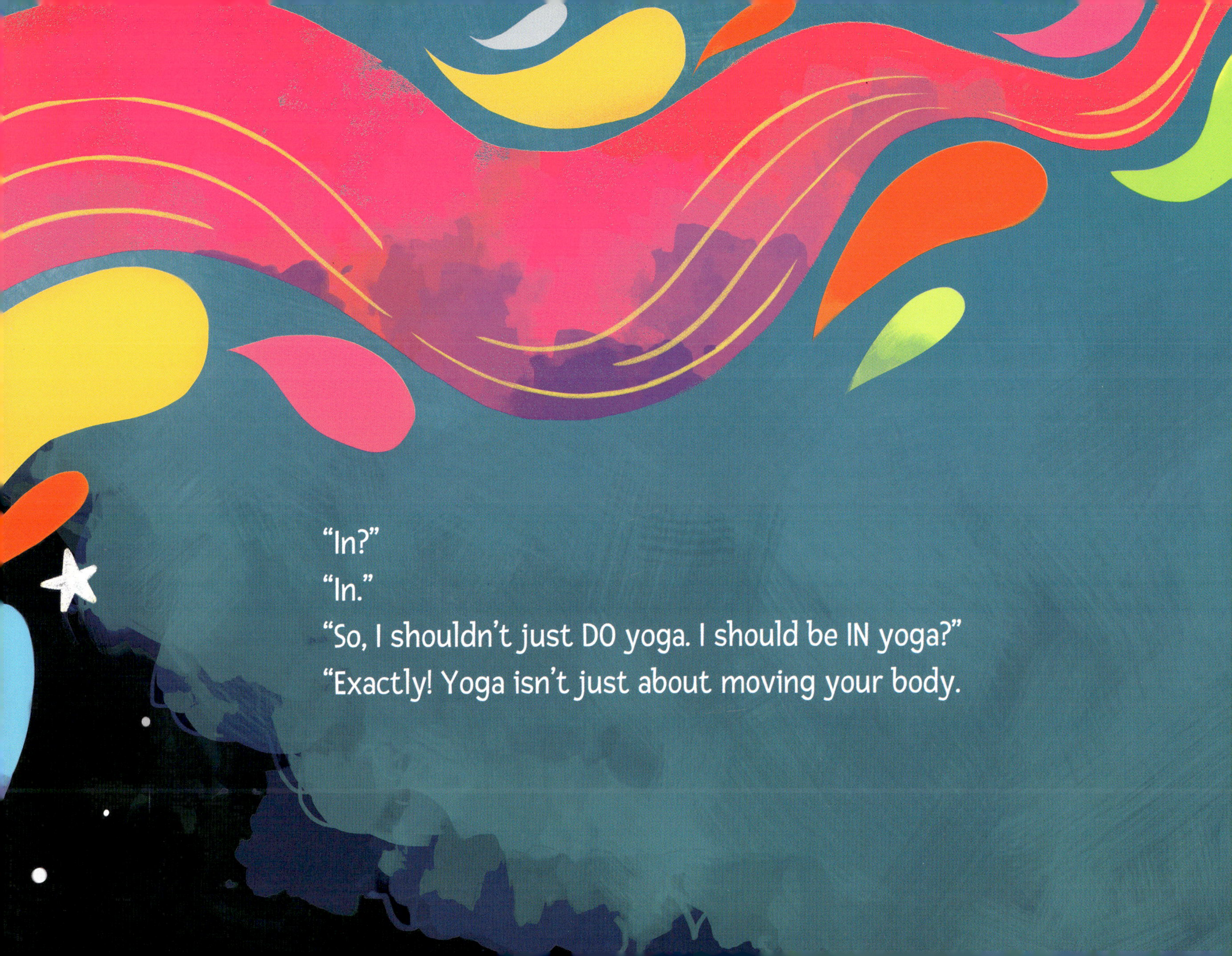

"In?"
"In."
"So, I shouldn't just DO yoga. I should be IN yoga?"
"Exactly! Yoga isn't just about moving your body.

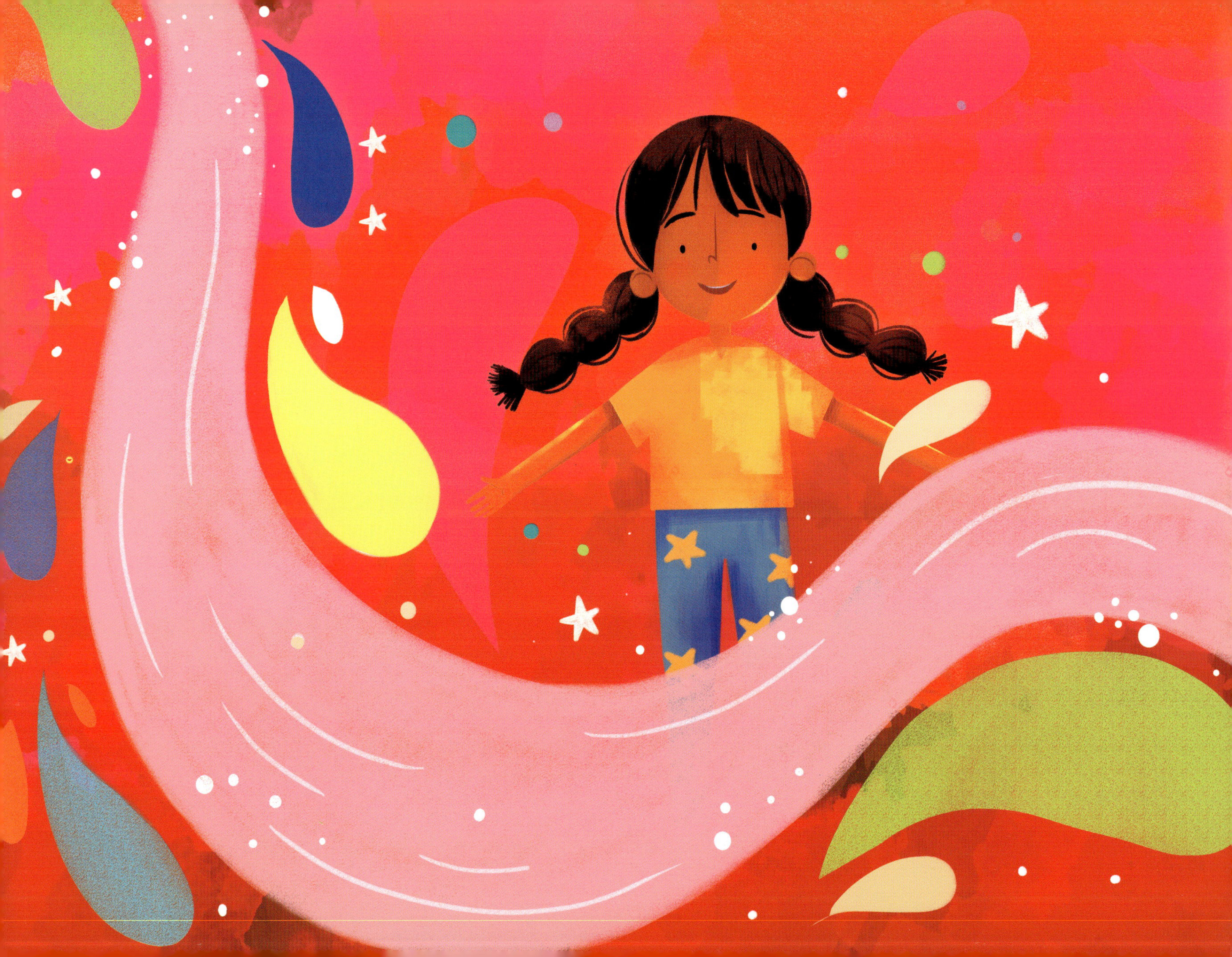

Yoga means union of your body, mind, emotions and energy. When they work together, anything you do such as sports, studying, reading etc your performance would be much better.

It's like a special science which shares ways for us to enJoy the world we live in, strengthen our body and boost our energy. It helps in taking care of ourselves and our surroundings well!

When you've got all that down, then you're in yoga."

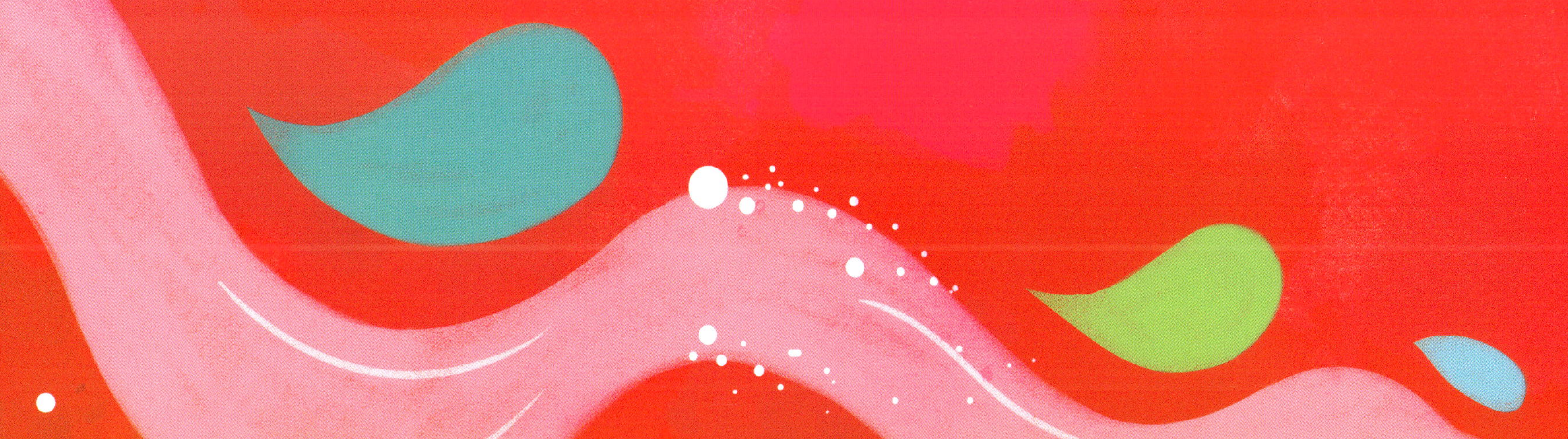

"But, how does being in yoga help me?"

"Yoga is like a superpower! It works on all levels.

Doing different poses called asanas, can make your body feel refreshed. Combine that with meditation and you have a clear mind! And a clear mind means relaxed emotions. On top of this, having fresh and colourful foods will recharge your batteries. When you put all of this together, you can feel your very best and stay better connected to yourself and everything around you."

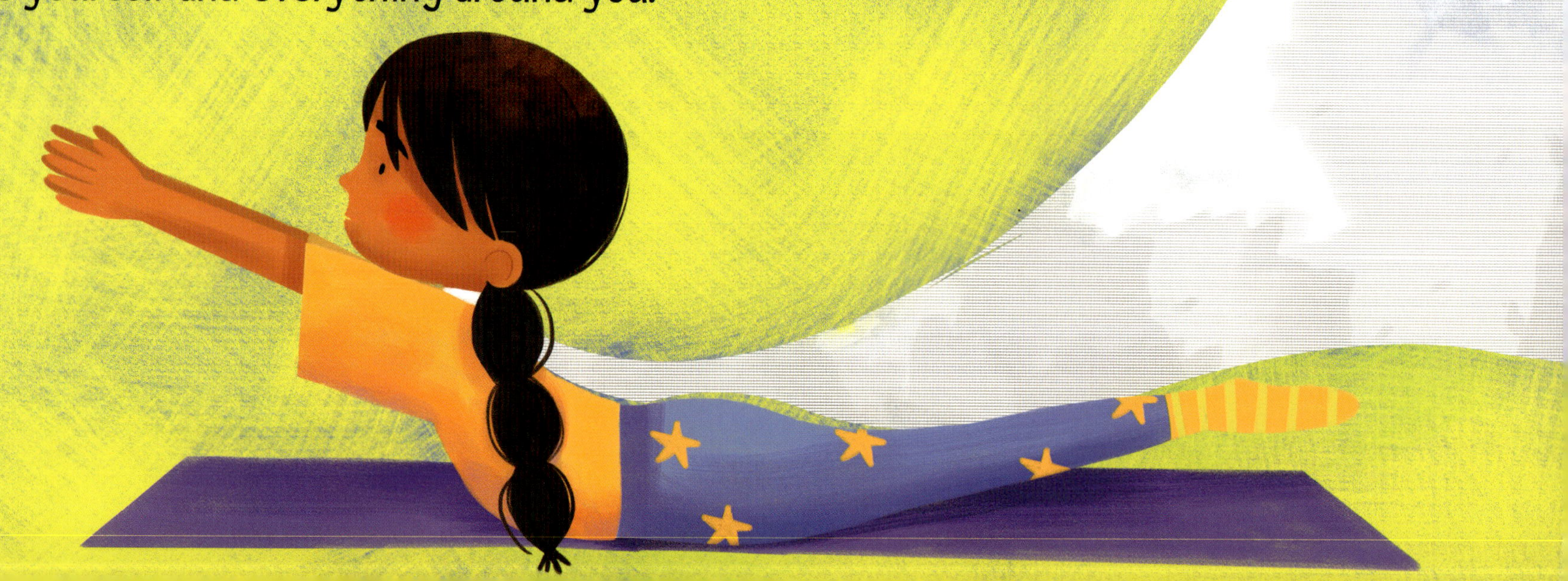

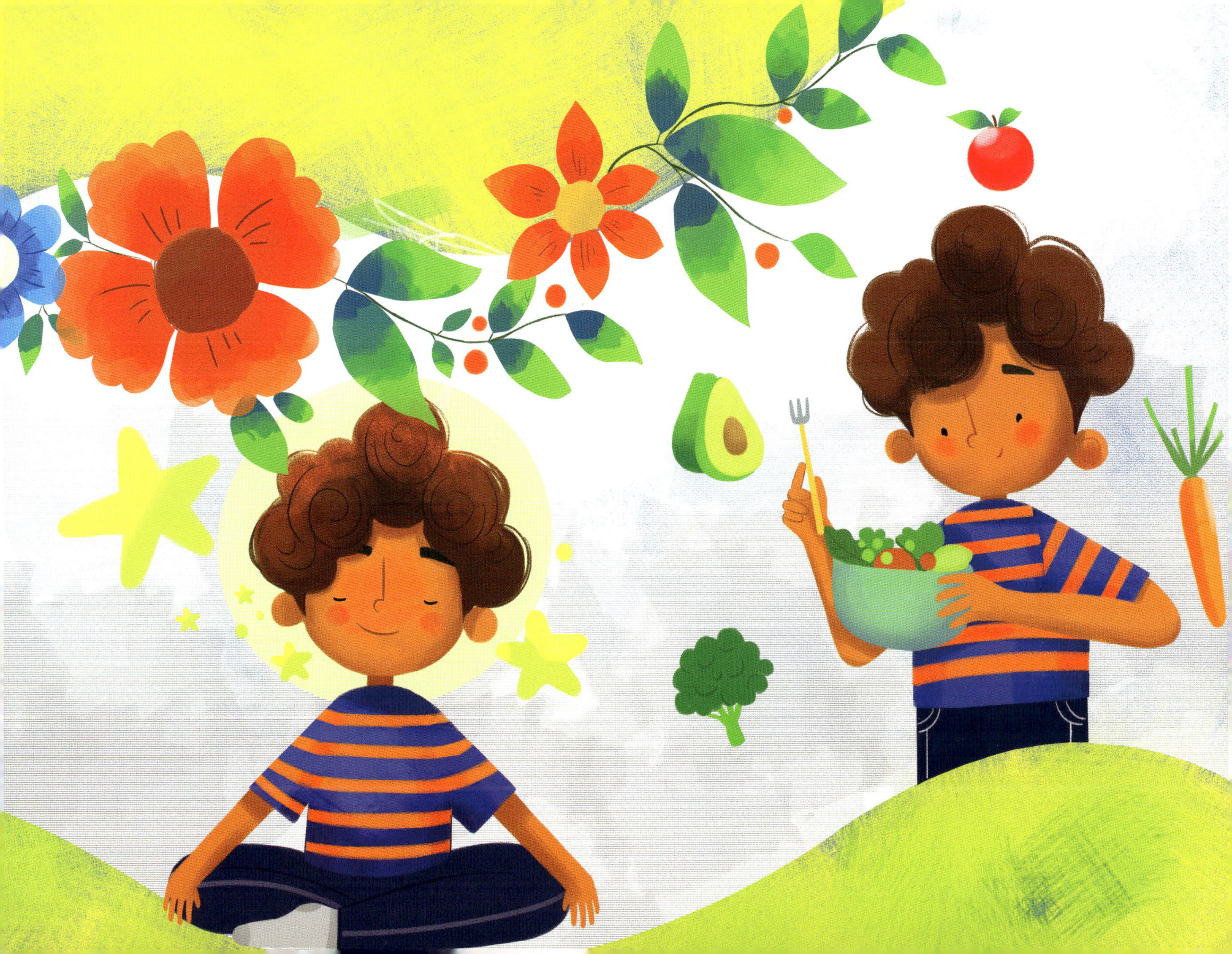

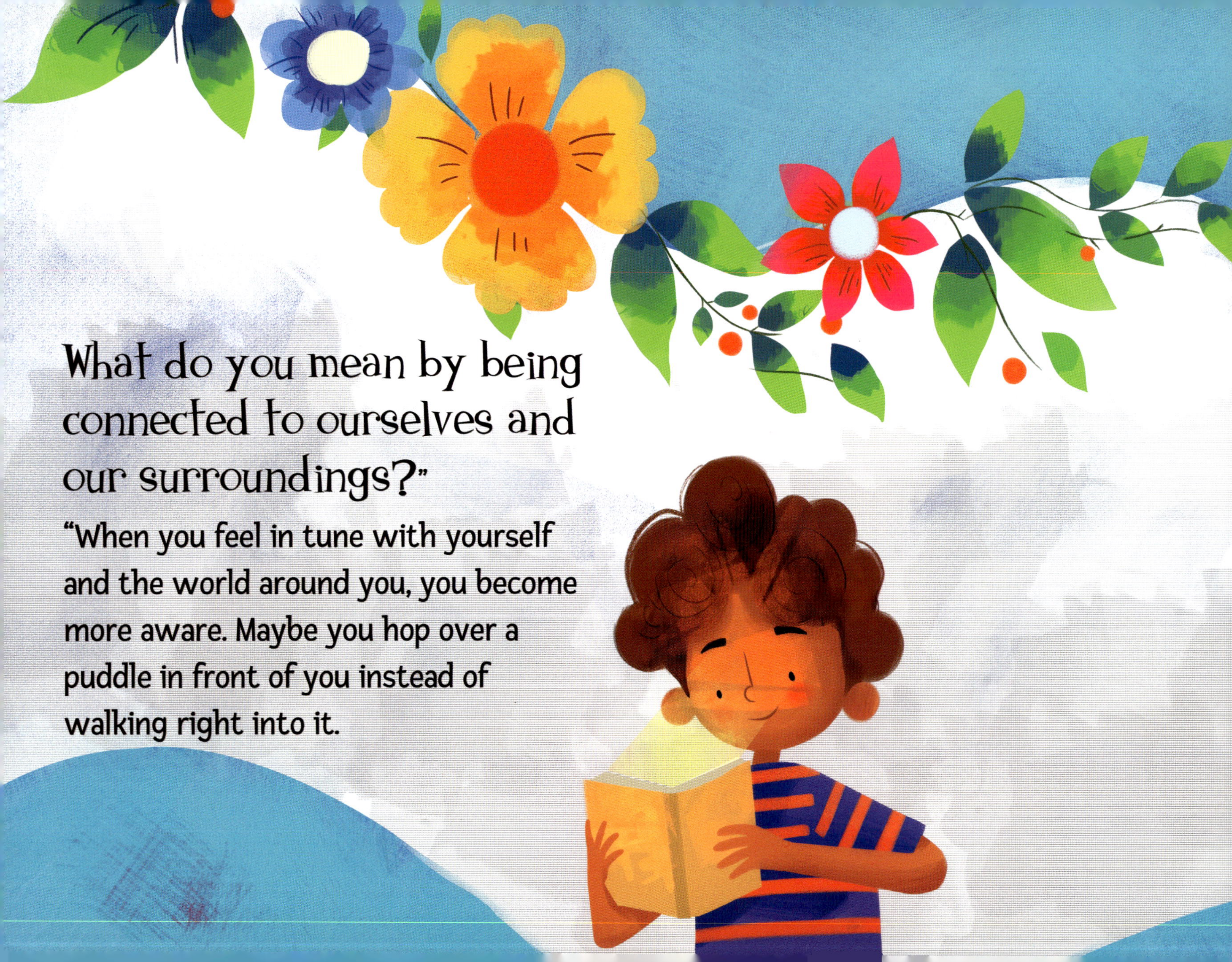

What do you mean by being connected to ourselves and our surroundings?"

"When you feel in tune with yourself and the world around you, you become more aware. Maybe you hop over a puddle in front of you instead of walking right into it.

Or your focus while reading gets better. You can catch a ball someone throws at you unexpectedly.

You may also be able to feel and express your emotions more calmly."

"Wow, this is quite interesting! I'm curious, who found out about yoga in the beginning?"

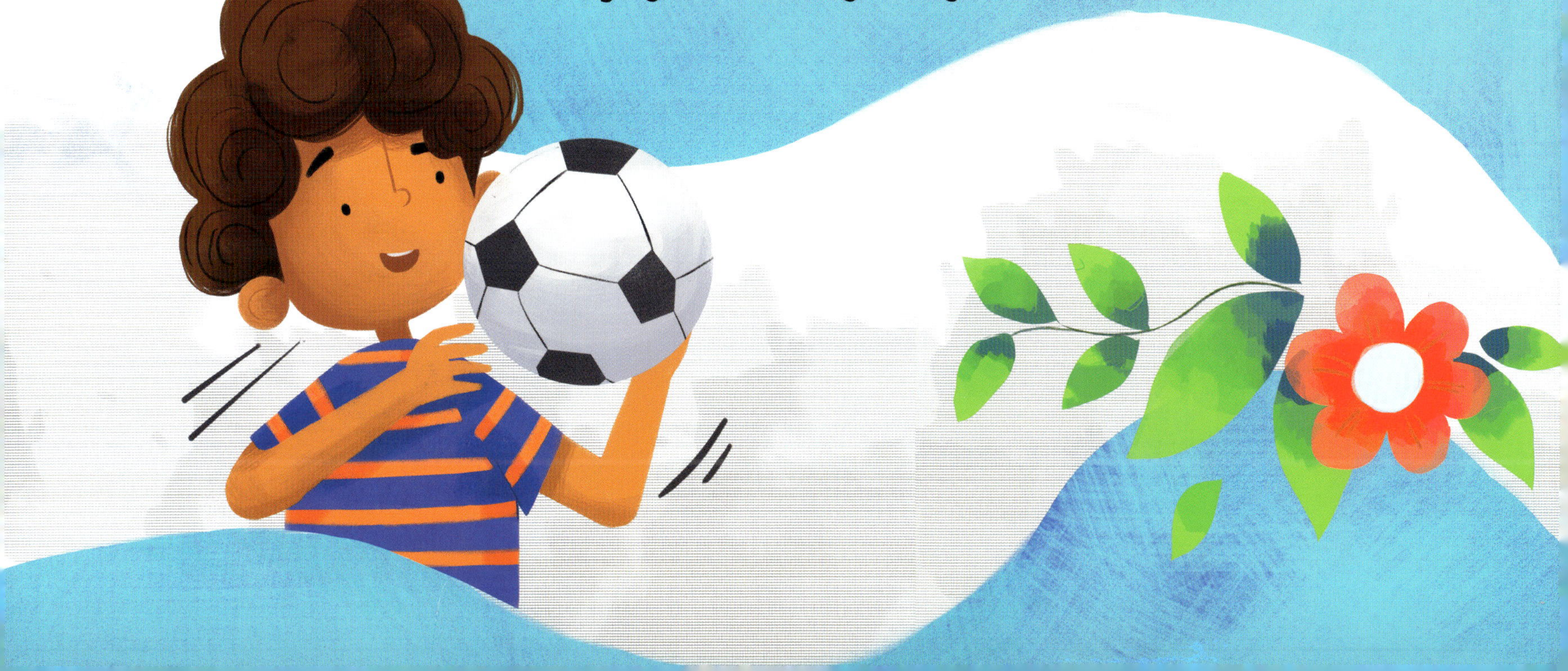

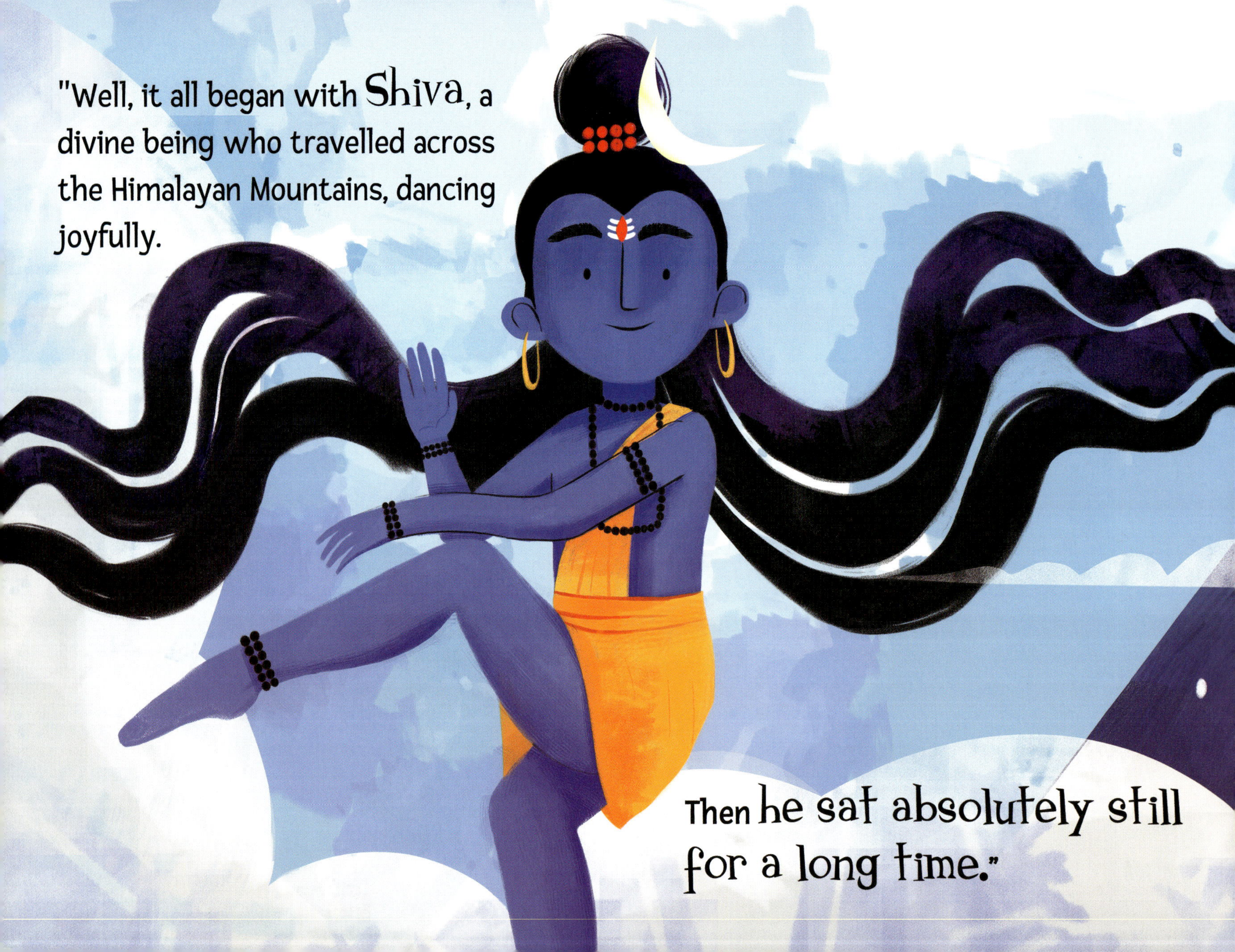

"Well, it all began with Shiva, a divine being who travelled across the Himalayan Mountains, dancing joyfully.

Then he sat absolutely still for a long time."

Did You Know?

Shiva has more than a thousand names! They all stem from the different qualities that Shiva is known for. He also has a family — a wife named Parvati and two kids, Kartikeya and Ganesha.

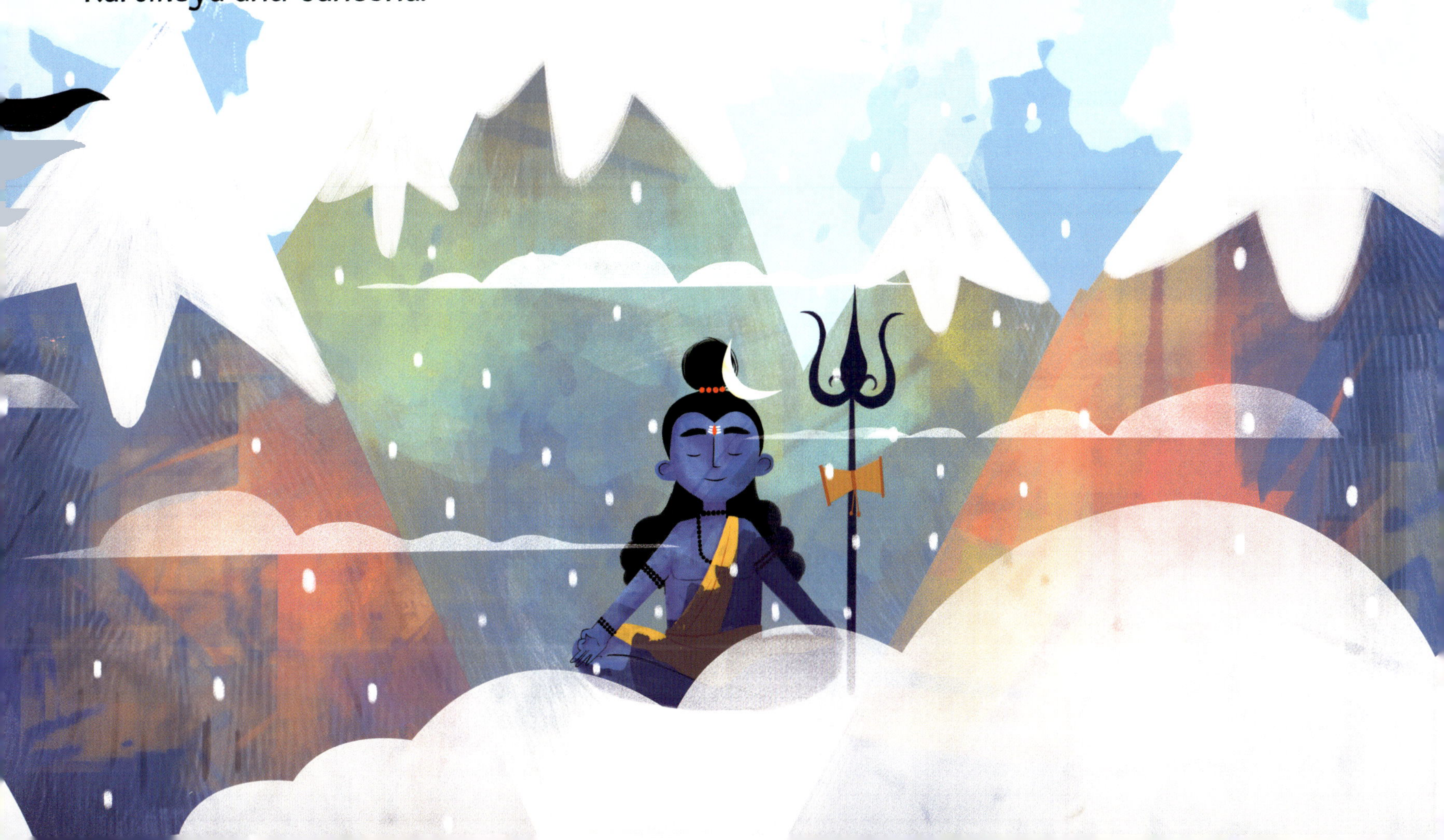

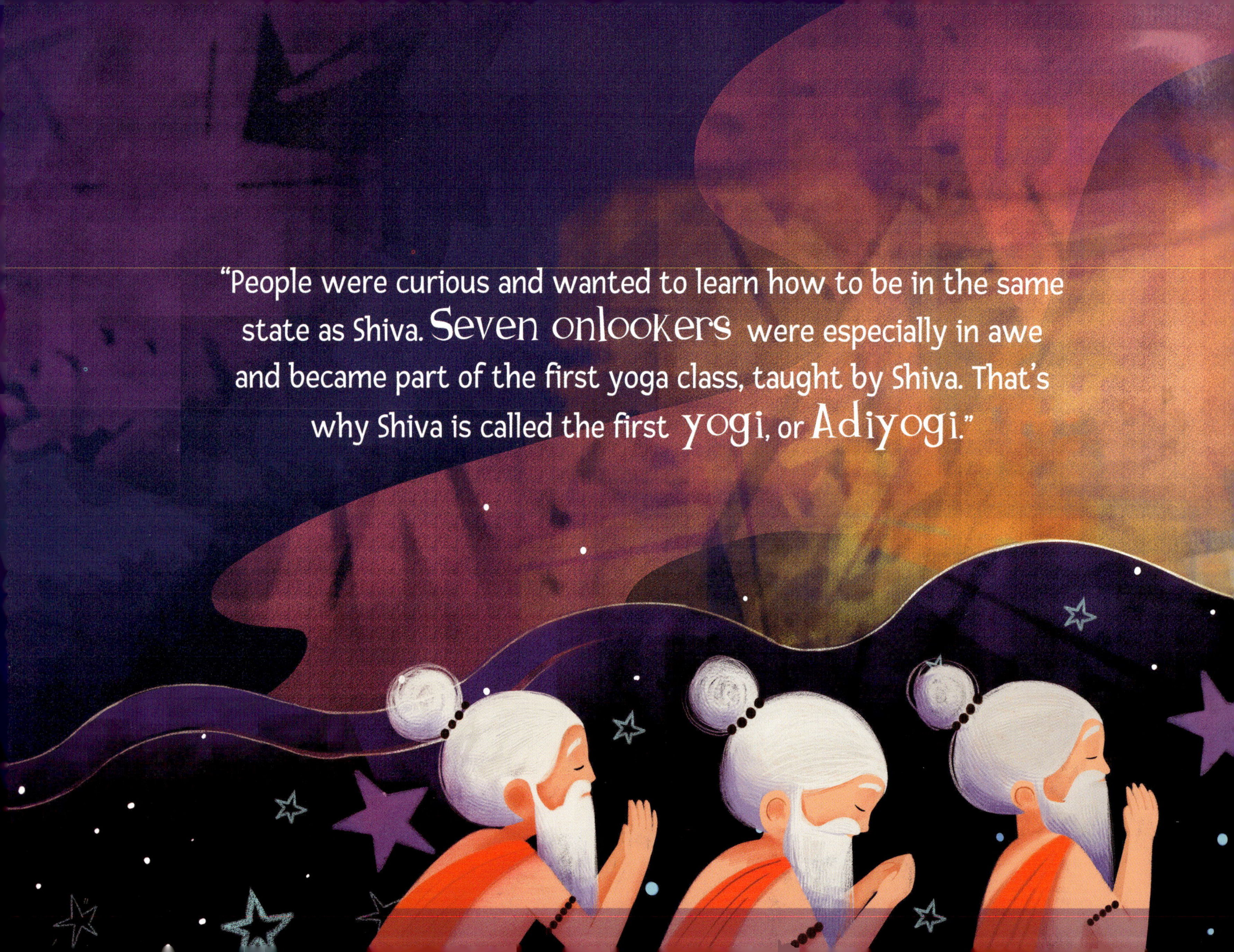

"People were curious and wanted to learn how to be in the same state as Shiva. Seven onlookers were especially in awe and became part of the first yoga class, taught by Shiva. That's why Shiva is called the first yogi, or Adiyogi."

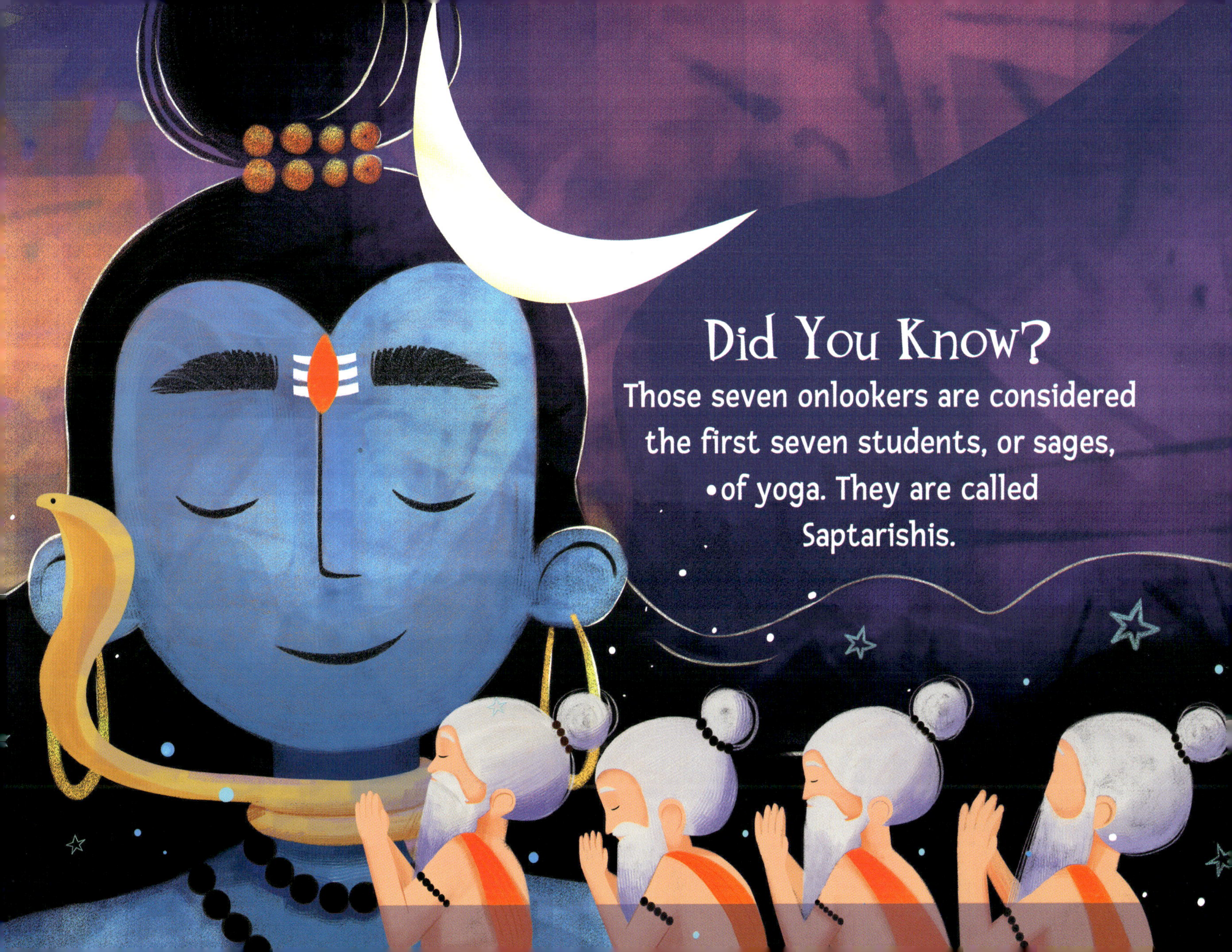
Did You Know?
Those seven onlookers are considered
the first seven students, or sages,
•of yoga. They are called
Saptarishis.

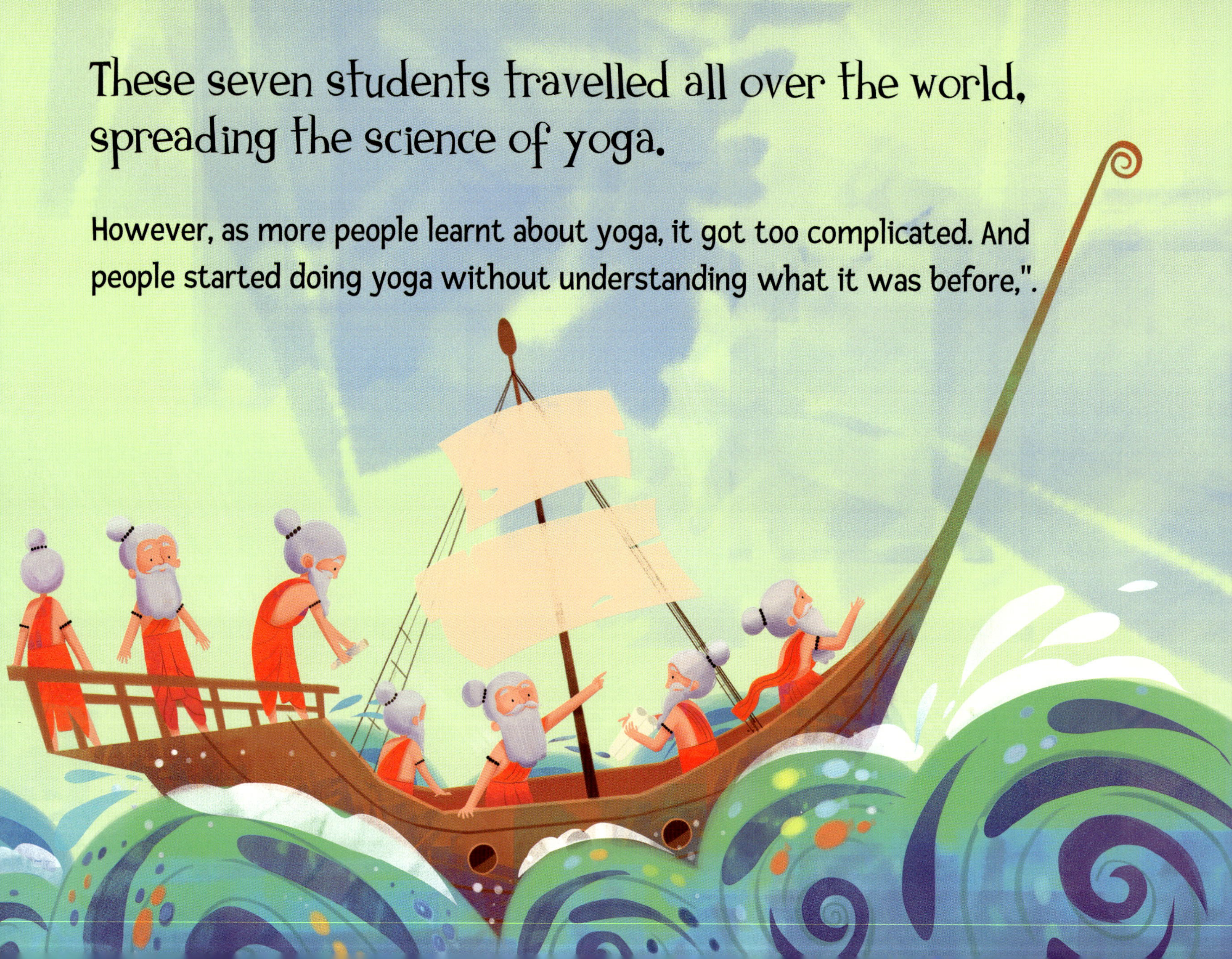

These seven students travelled all over the world, spreading the science of yoga.

However, as more people learnt about yoga, it got too complicated. And people started doing yoga without understanding what it was before,".

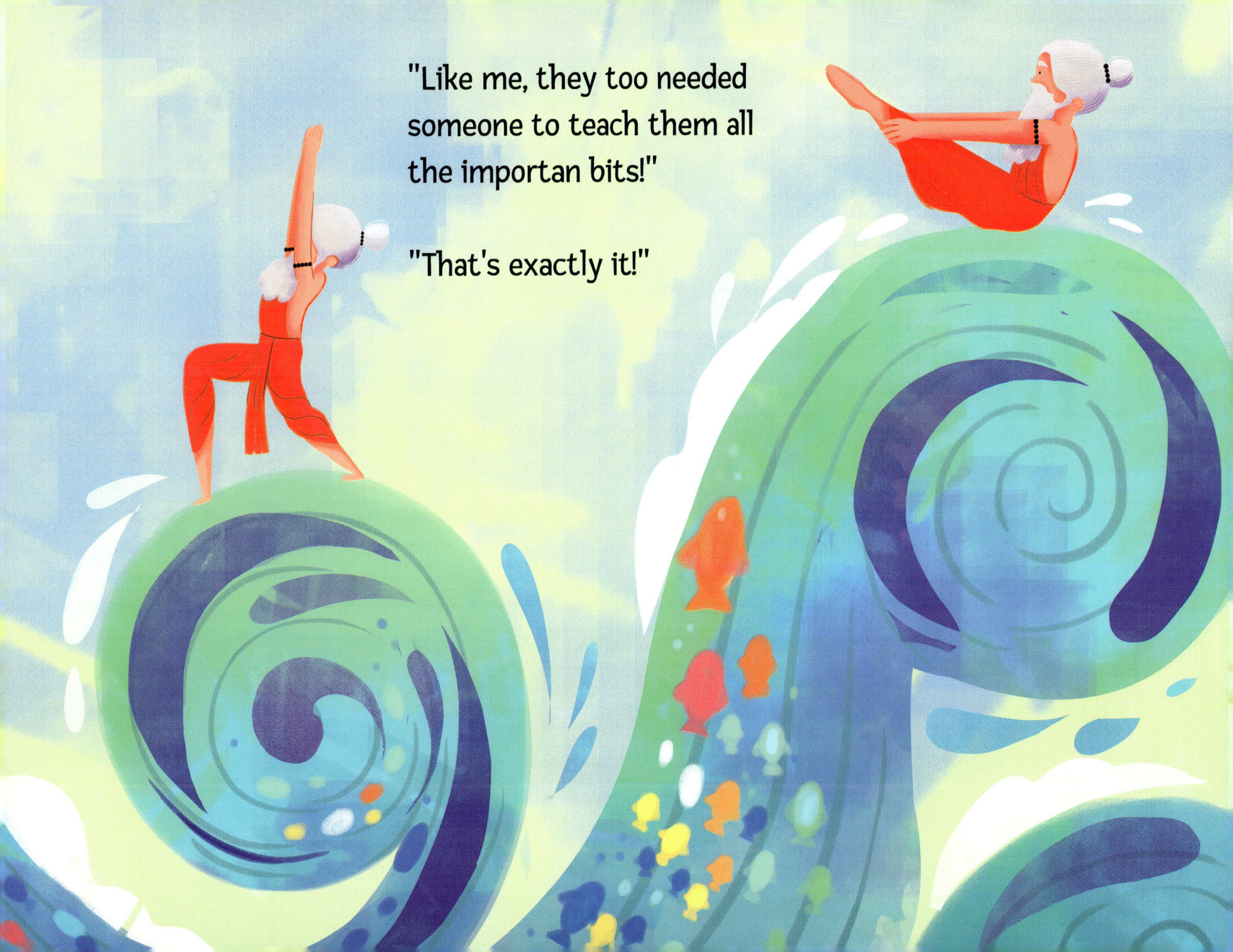

"Like me, they too needed someone to teach them all the importan bits!"

"That's exactly it!"

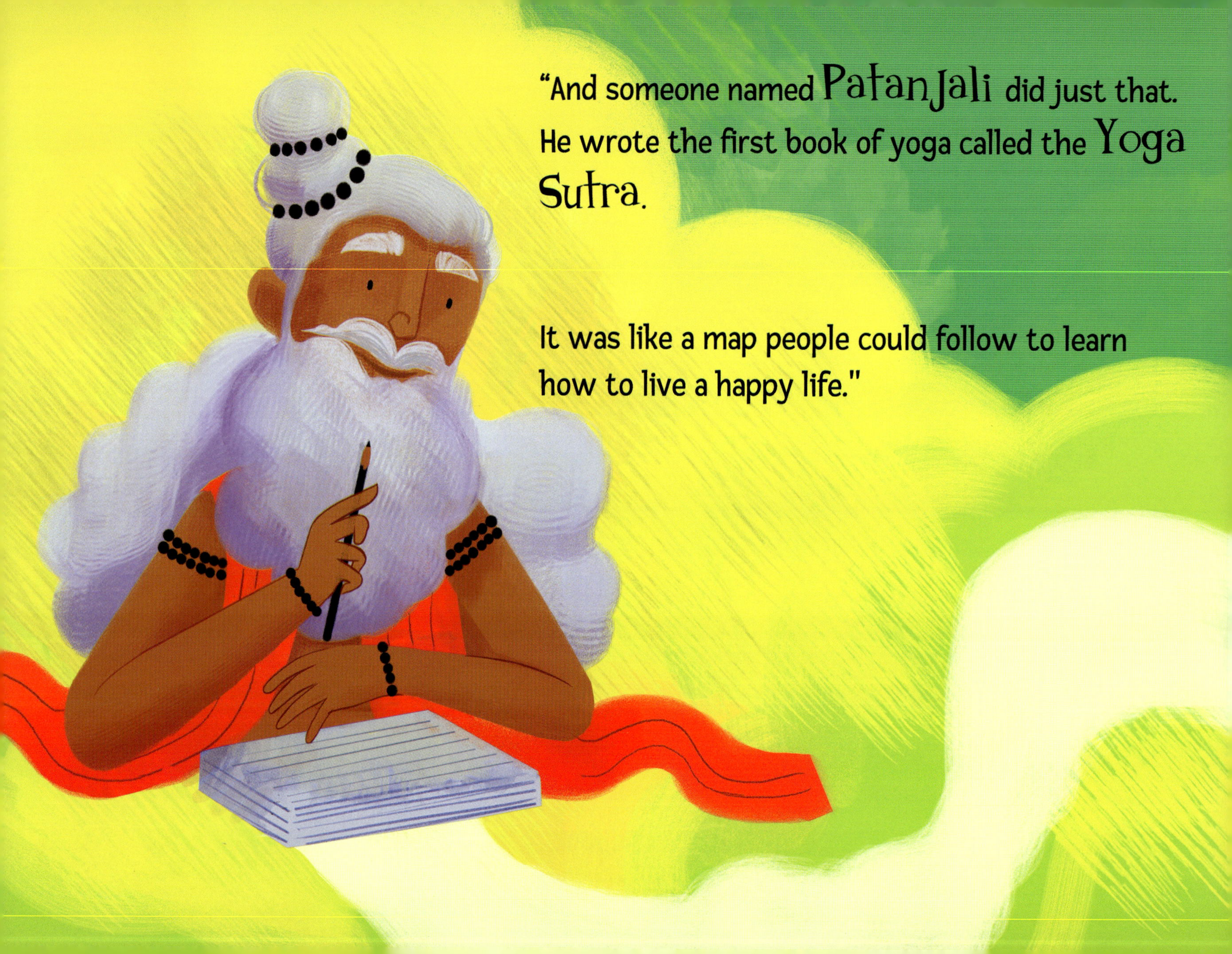

"And someone named PatanJali did just that. He wrote the first book of yoga called the Yoga Sutra.

It was like a map people could follow to learn how to live a happy life."

Did You Know?

Patanjali is known as the father of modern yoga. Some consider him to be a genius who wrote the entire Yoga Sutra. While others say that the Yoga Sutra took centuries to write and Patanjali is really different people all writing under the same name.

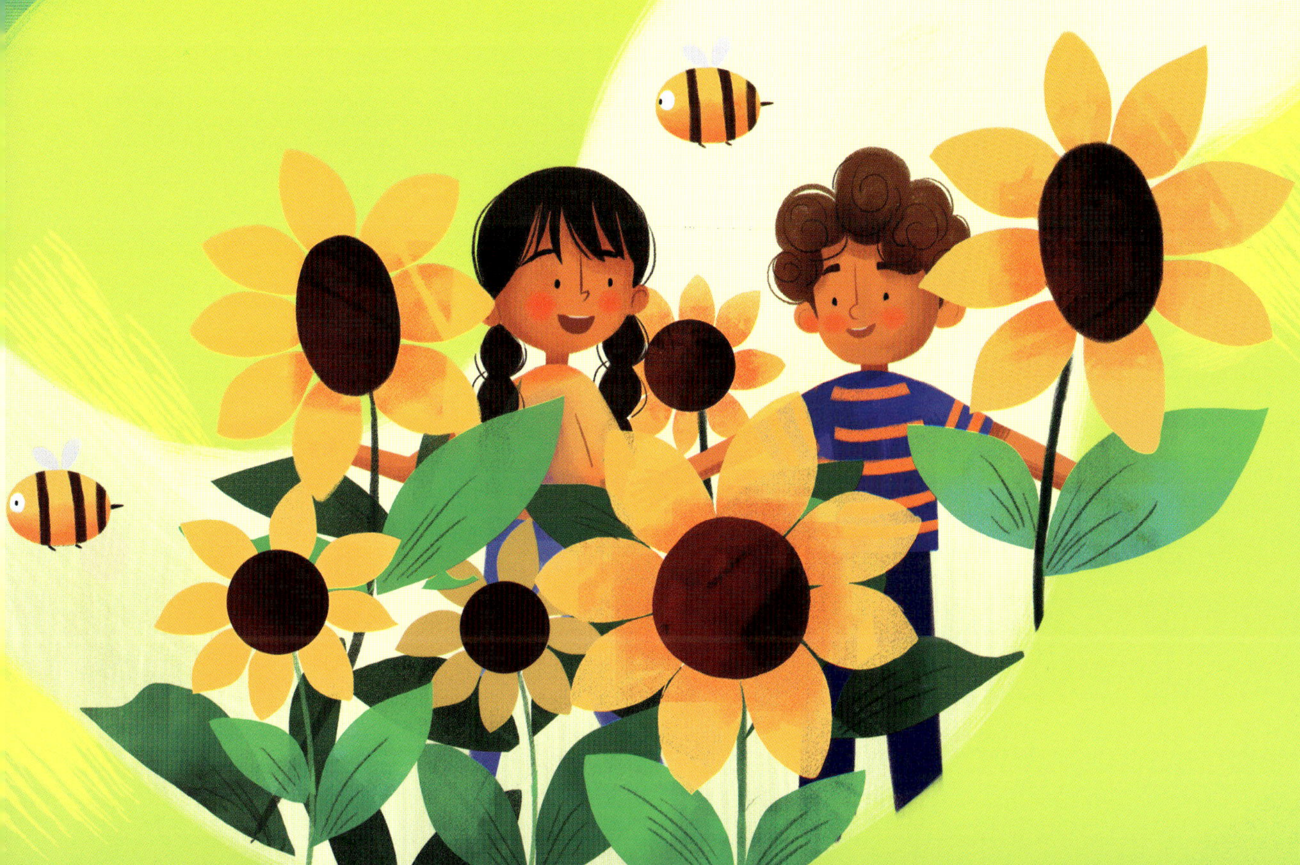

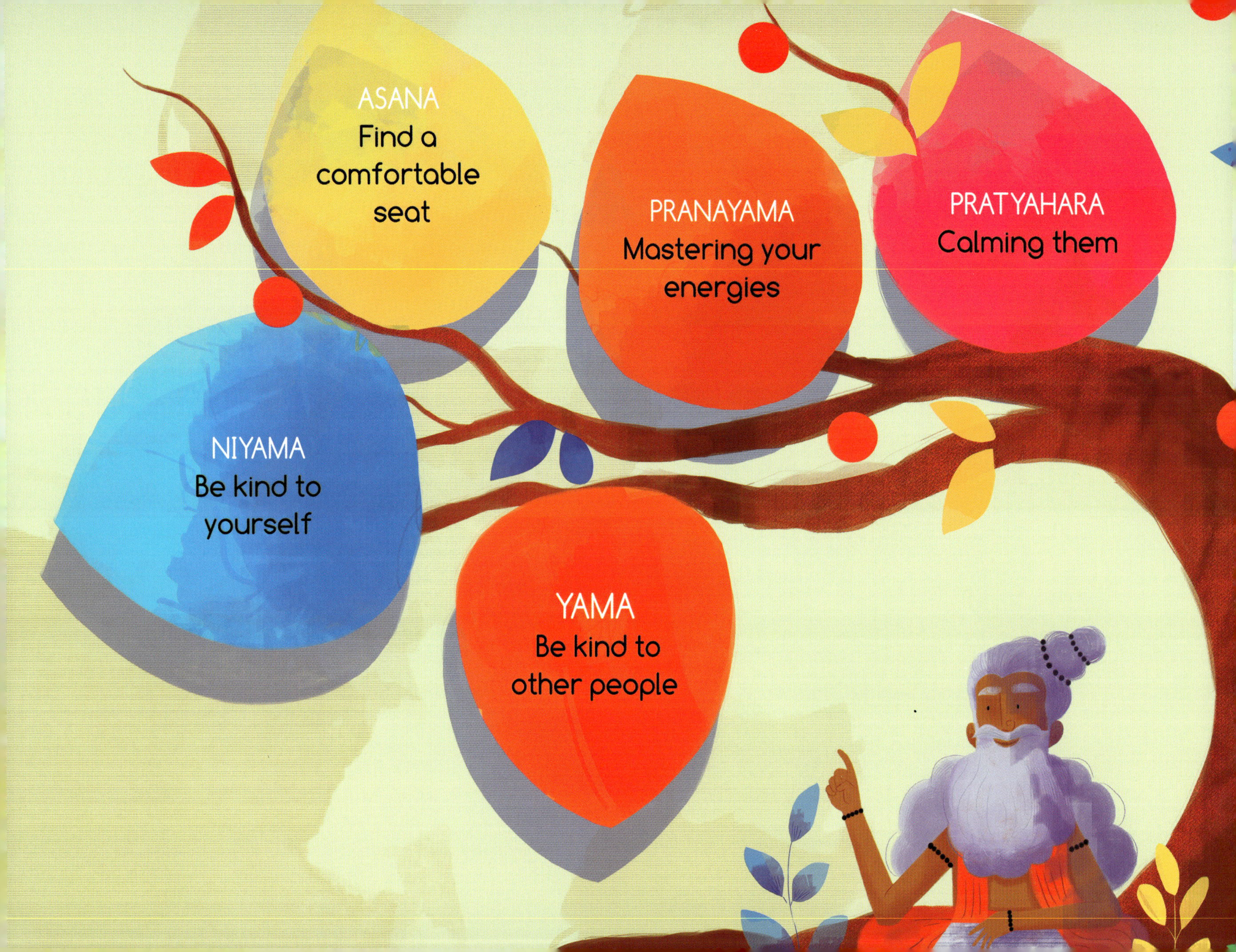

ASANA
Find a comfortable seat

PRANAYAMA
Mastering your energies

PRATYAHARA
Calming them

NIYAMA
Be kind to yourself

YAMA
Be kind to other people

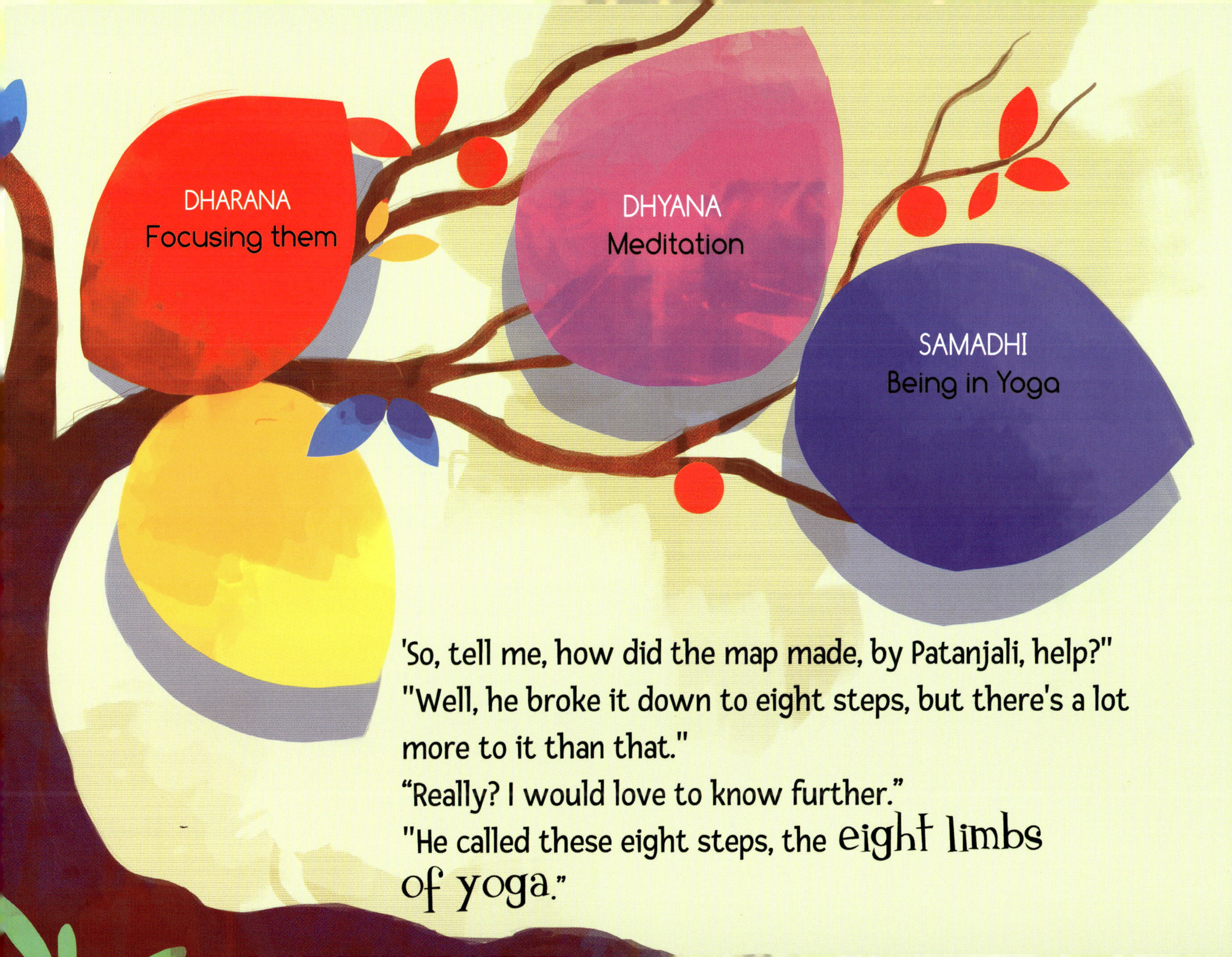

'So, tell me, how did the map made, by Patanjali, help?"
"Well, he broke it down to eight steps, but there's a lot more to it than that."
"Really? I would love to know further."
"He called these eight steps, the eight limbs of yoga."

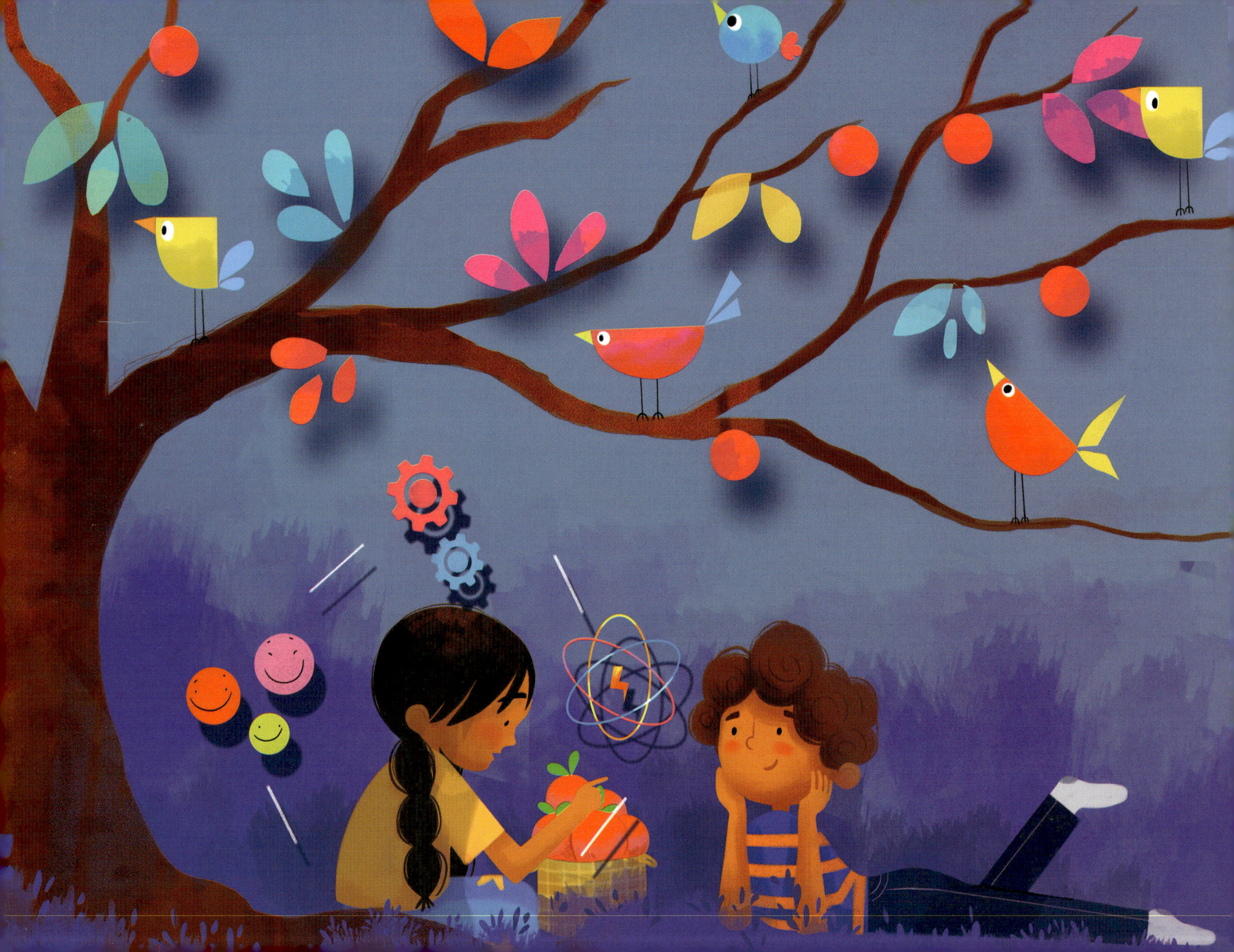

"Remember, you can't do these steps just once. You have to do them over and over until you really get it. And you also have to concentrate on a few other things at the same time."

"Oh! that's deep! So, to become a super-human, do I need to learn the basics of mind, body, energy first?

Did You Know?

The body, the mind, your emotions, and your energy are considered the four fundamental types of yoga. Some people like to focus more on their body when they do yoga (that's karma yoga). While some people like to work on their internal energies (that's kriya yoga), others like to focus more on their emotions (that's bhakti yoga), and still others like to concentrate more on their energy (gnana yoga). It doesn't matter which you lean on most, but a true yogi must learn how to use all four.

"These elements tie the body and its layers! There are 5 sheaths or layers – one inside the other, called koshas."

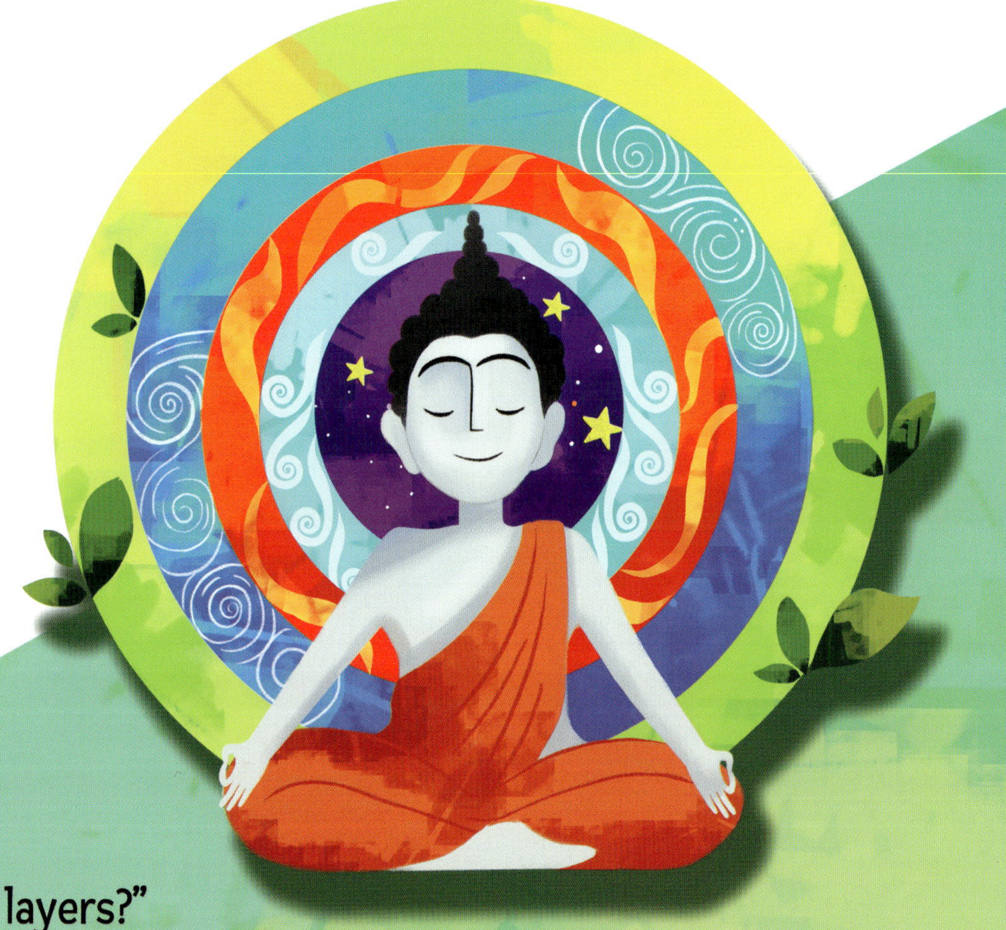

"Our body has five layers?"
"Yes! Let me tell you what they are! What is the first thing you see when you look at the mirror?" "Myself?"

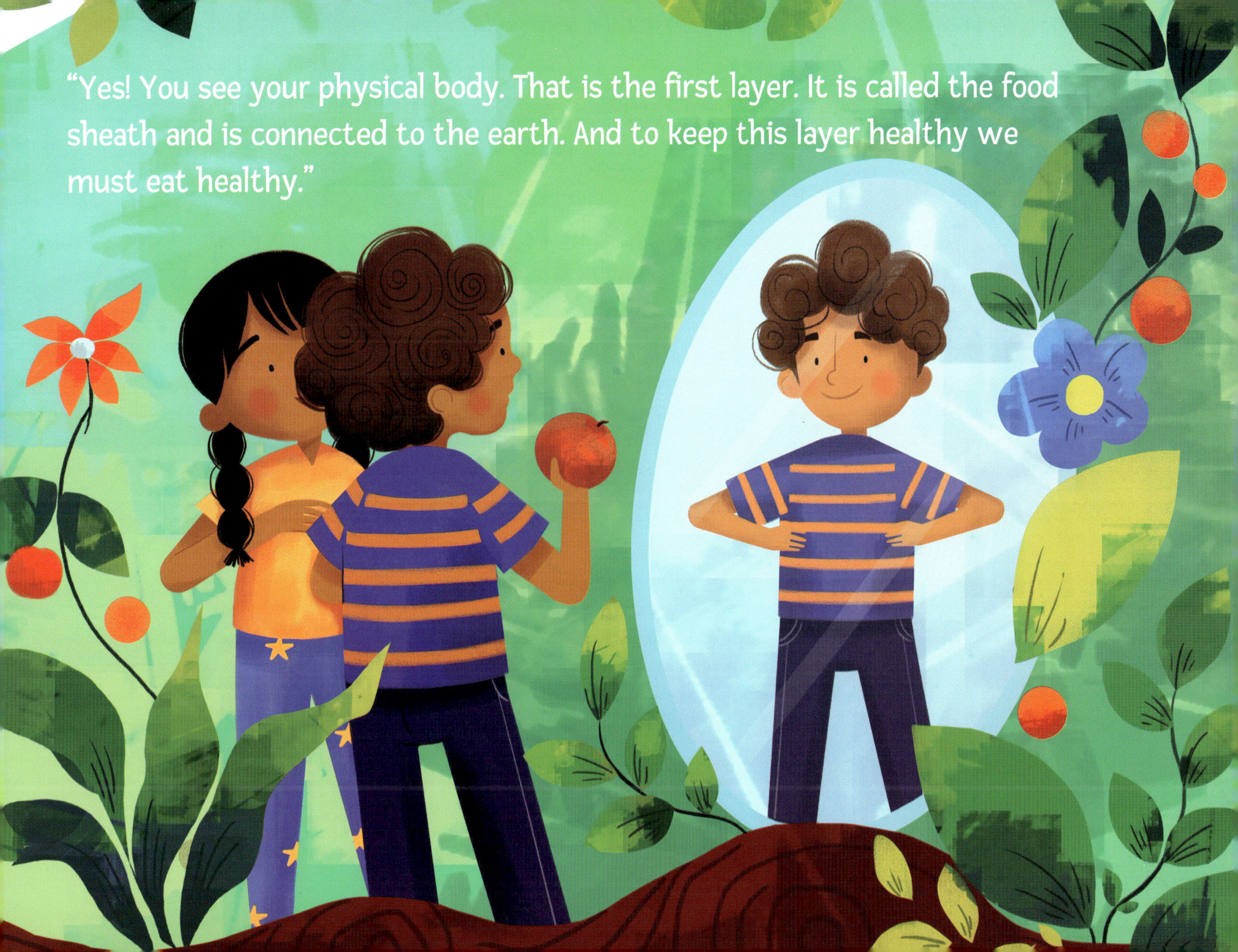
"Yes! You see your physical body. That is the first layer. It is called the food sheath and is connected to the earth. And to keep this layer healthy we must eat healthy."

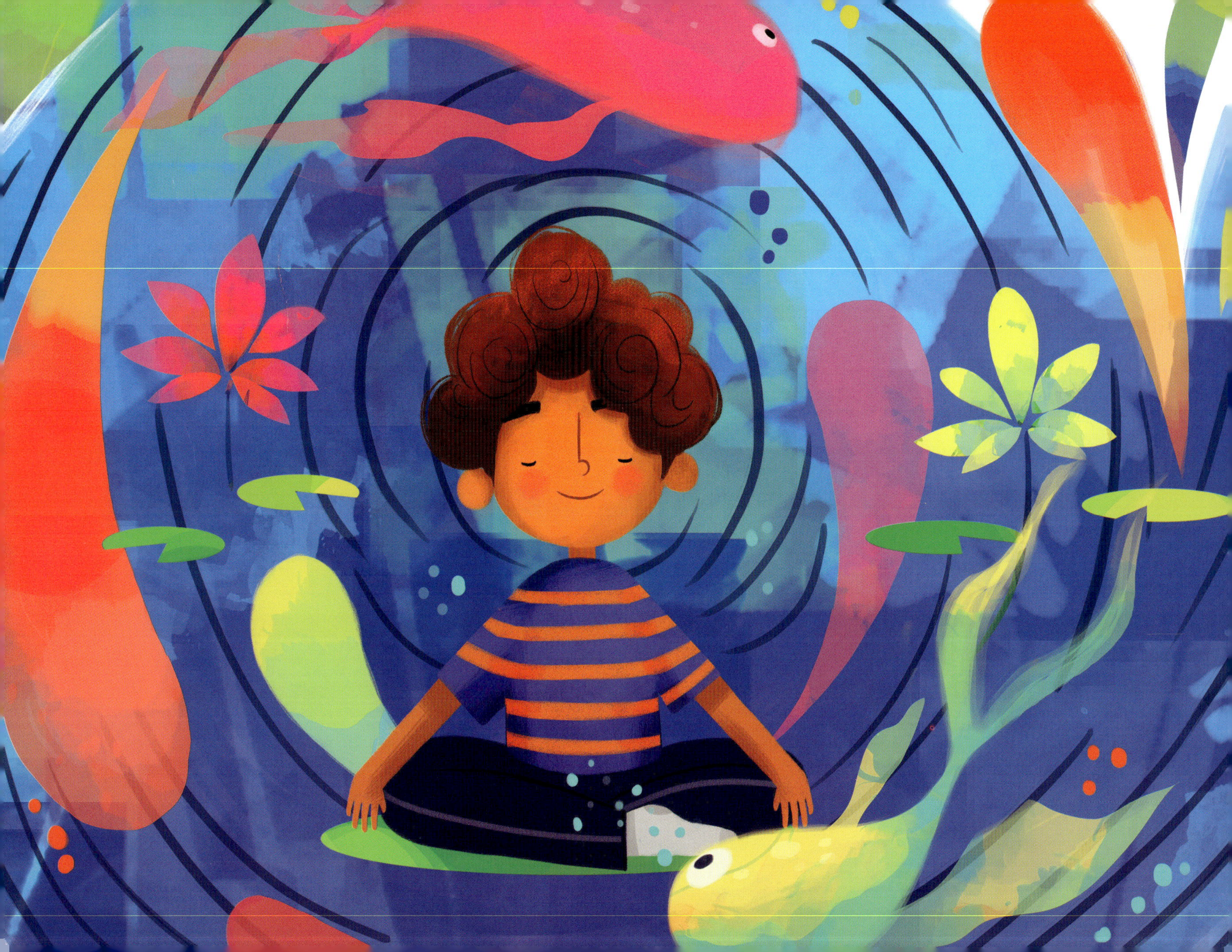

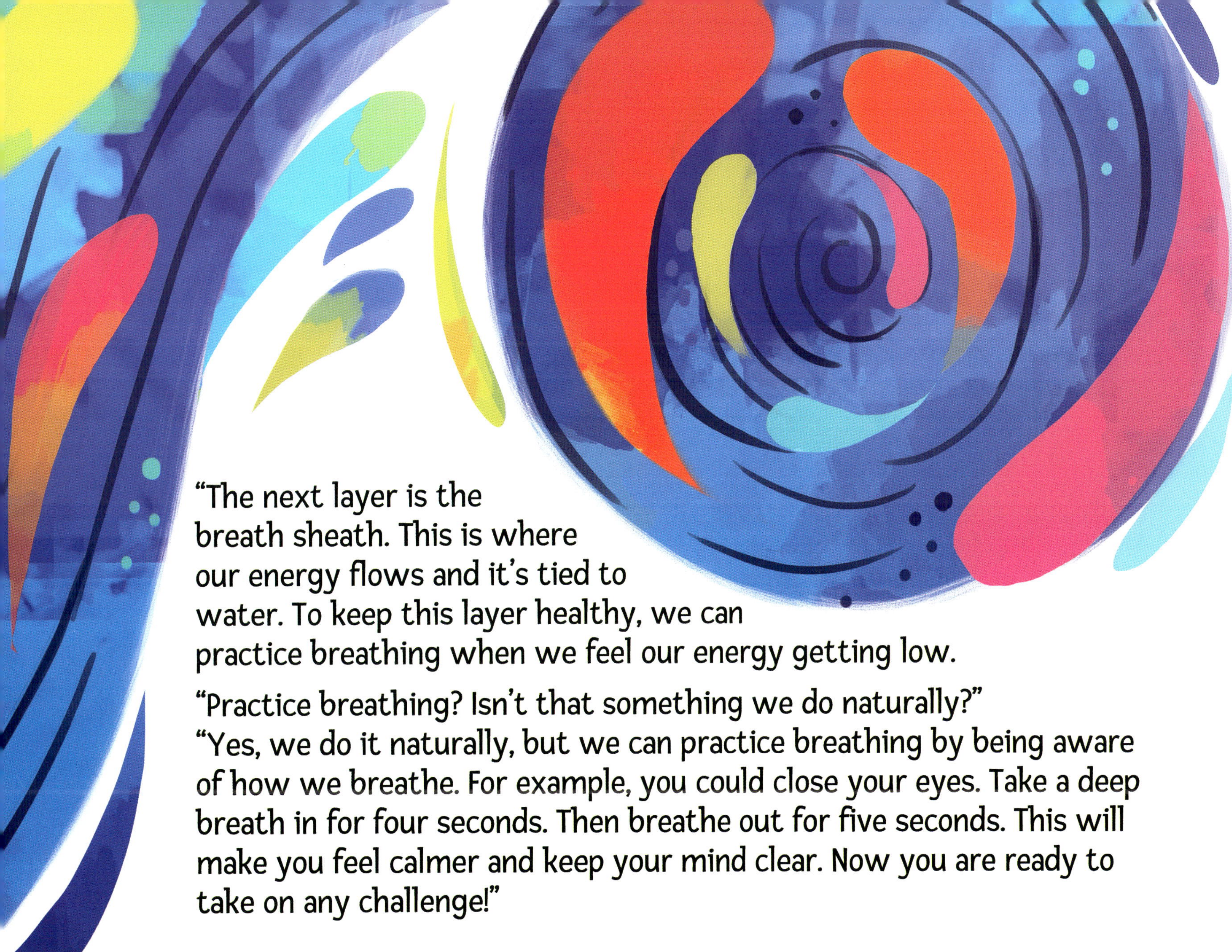

"The next layer is the breath sheath. This is where our energy flows and it's tied to water. To keep this layer healthy, we can practice breathing when we feel our energy getting low.

"Practice breathing? Isn't that something we do naturally?"
"Yes, we do it naturally, but we can practice breathing by being aware of how we breathe. For example, you could close your eyes. Take a deep breath in for four seconds. Then breathe out for five seconds. This will make you feel calmer and keep your mind clear. Now you are ready to take on any challenge!"

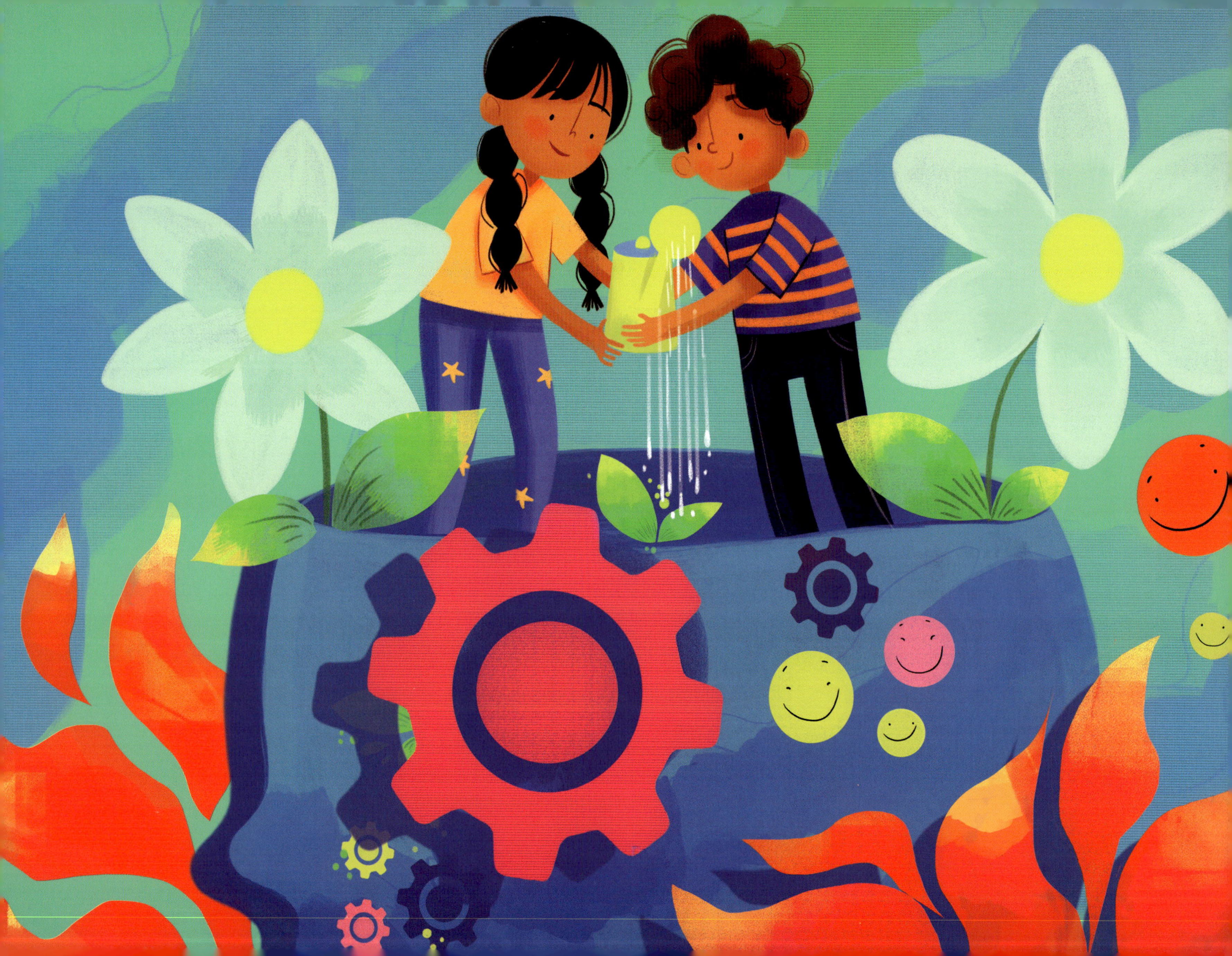

"Amazing!"

"Next, we have the mind sheath. This is the layer where our thoughts and emotions come from. It's tied to the fire element. To keep our mental sheath healthy, we should think positively!" "How will thinking positively help?"

"For example, you are experiencing an upsetting situation like missing out on playground time, or you were not able to finish a test the way you would've liked to. In situations like these, taking a deep breath and thinking something like - 'I can handle this' or 'I am happy, I am calm', can help you feel better."

"Really? I will have to try this the next time I am frustrated at not being able to score a goal."

"I think learning about the next layer will also help you." "For real? Then tell me quickly!"

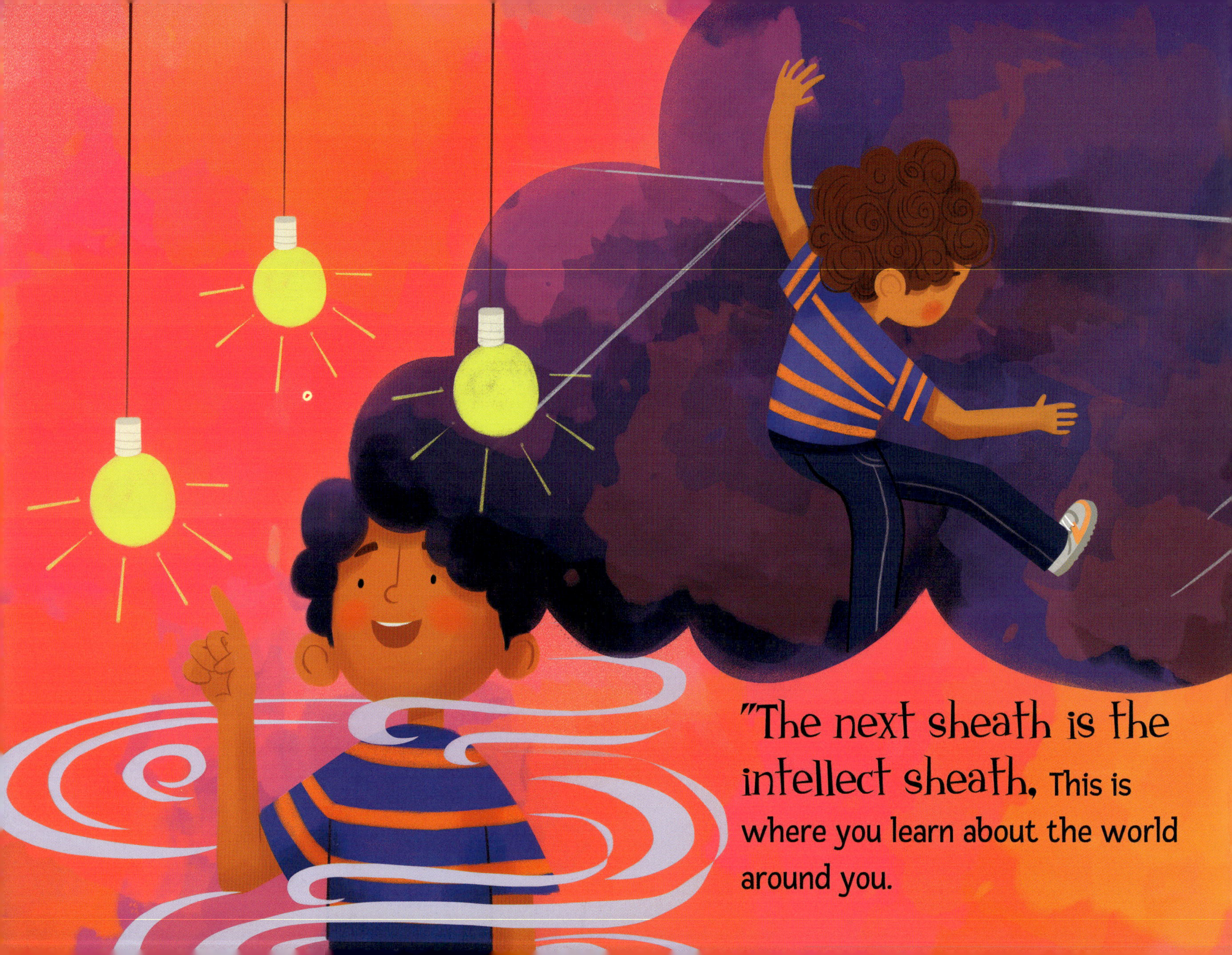
"The next sheath is the intellect sheath. This is where you learn about the world around you.

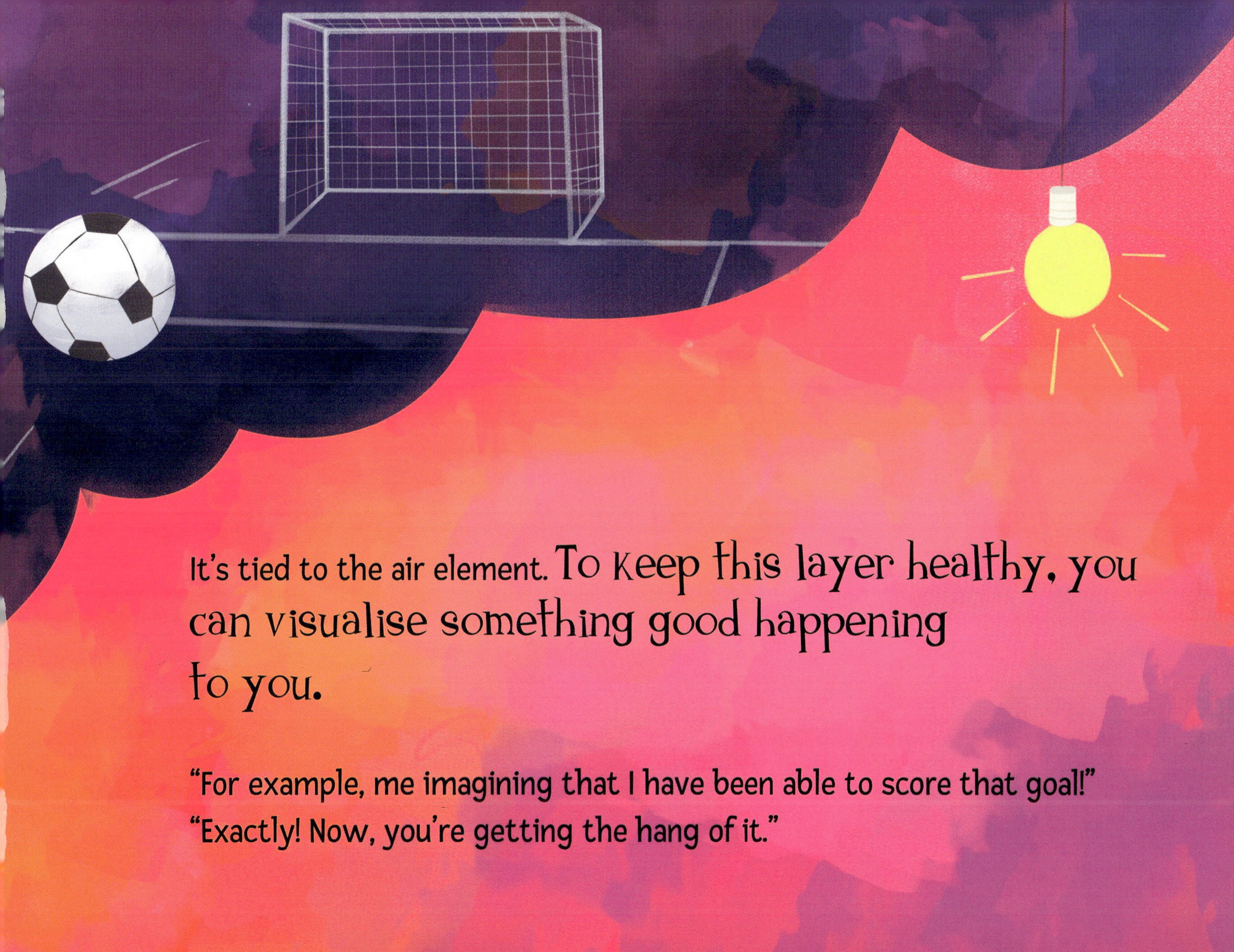

It's tied to the air element. To keep this layer healthy, you can visualise something good happening to you.

"For example, me imagining that I have been able to score that goal!"
"Exactly! Now, you're getting the hang of it."

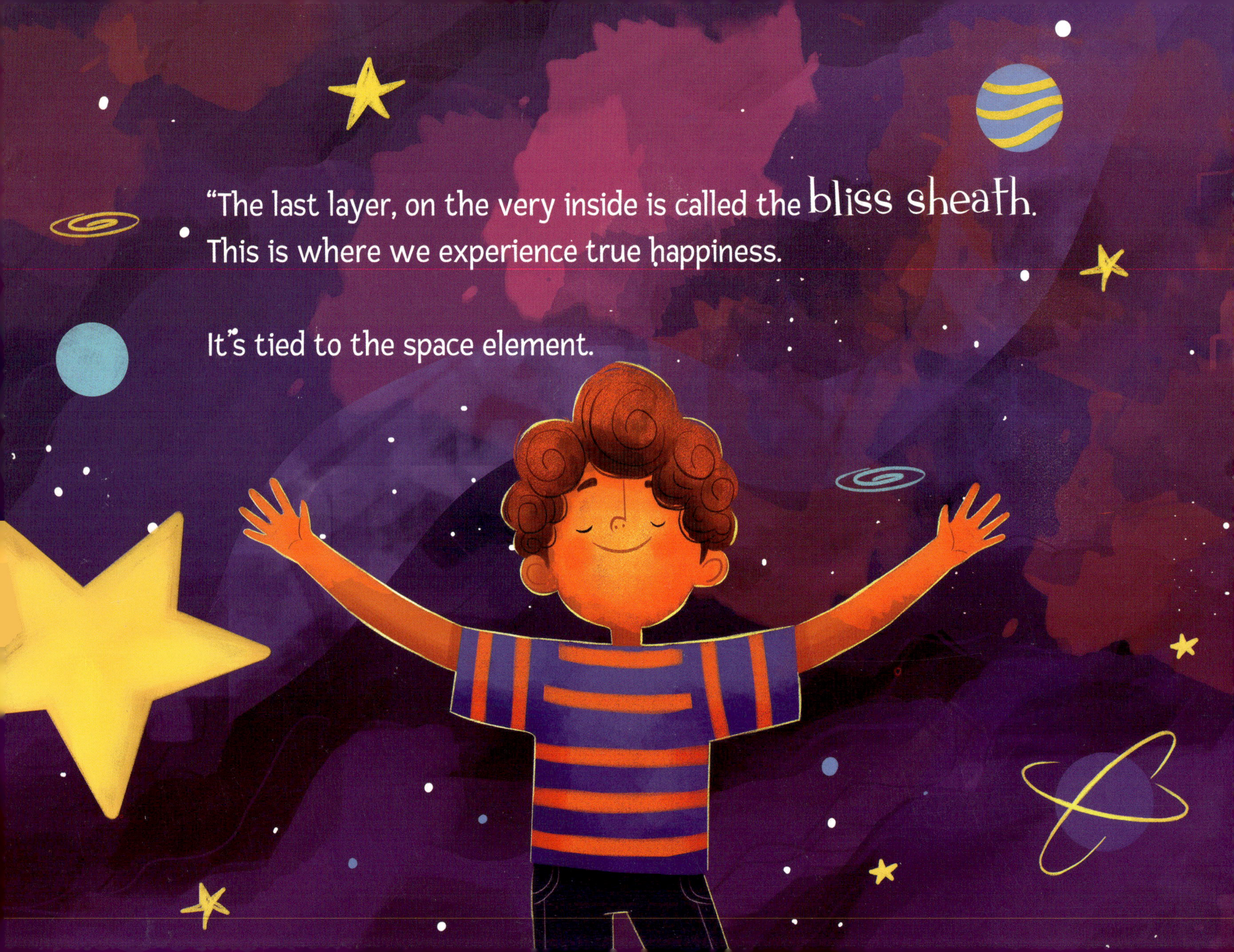

"The last layer, on the very inside is called the bliss sheath. This is where we experience true happiness.

It's tied to the space element.

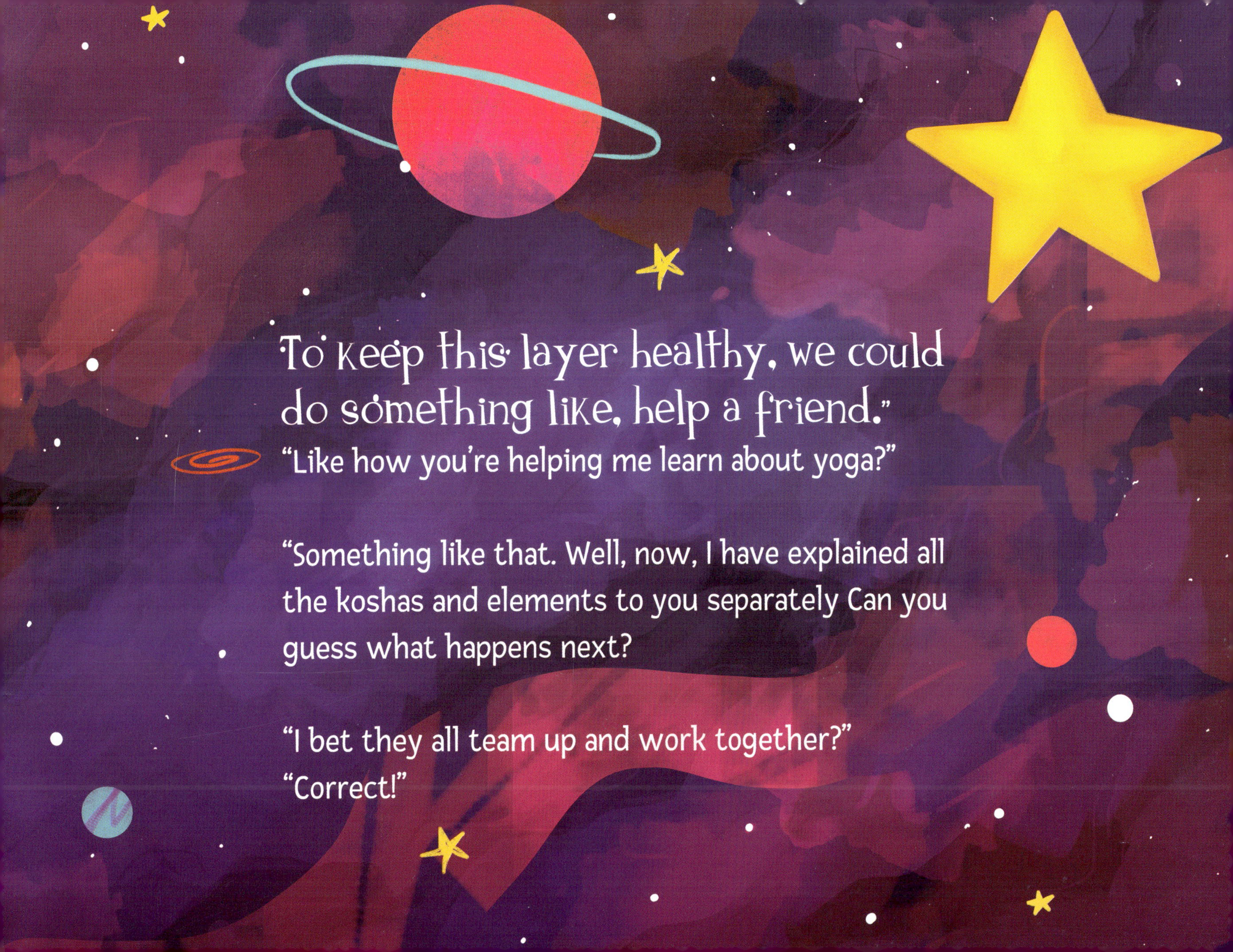

To keep this layer healthy, we could do something like, help a friend."
"Like how you're helping me learn about yoga?"

"Something like that. Well, now, I have explained all the koshas and elements to you separately Can you guess what happens next?

"I bet they all team up and work together?"
"Correct!"

"Are we ready to do yoga now?"
"I've just one last thing to tell you."
"I'm all ears!"
"It's about your chakras."

"Chakras?"

"Your chakras are like
wheels that spin and
pull energy into your
body.

If those wheels spin too fast or too
slow, then there's a problem.

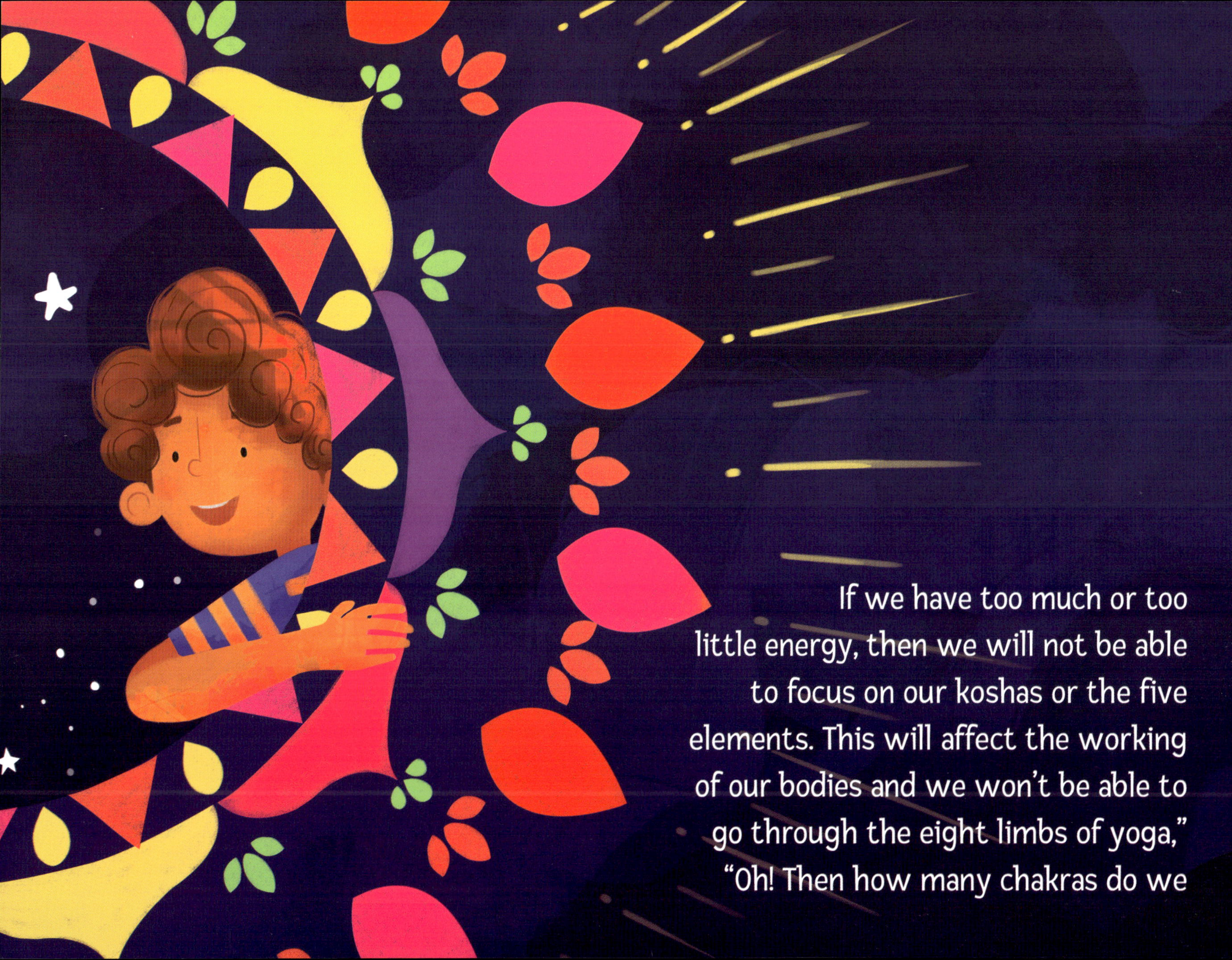

If we have too much or too
little energy, then we will not be able
to focus on our koshas or the five
elements. This will affect the working
of our bodies and we won't be able to
go through the eight limbs of yoga,"
"Oh! Then how many chakras do we

"Well, there are over 100, but there are seven that we focus on the most.

The first chakra is at the bottom of your spine.

It's the one that balances who you are and how you got here."

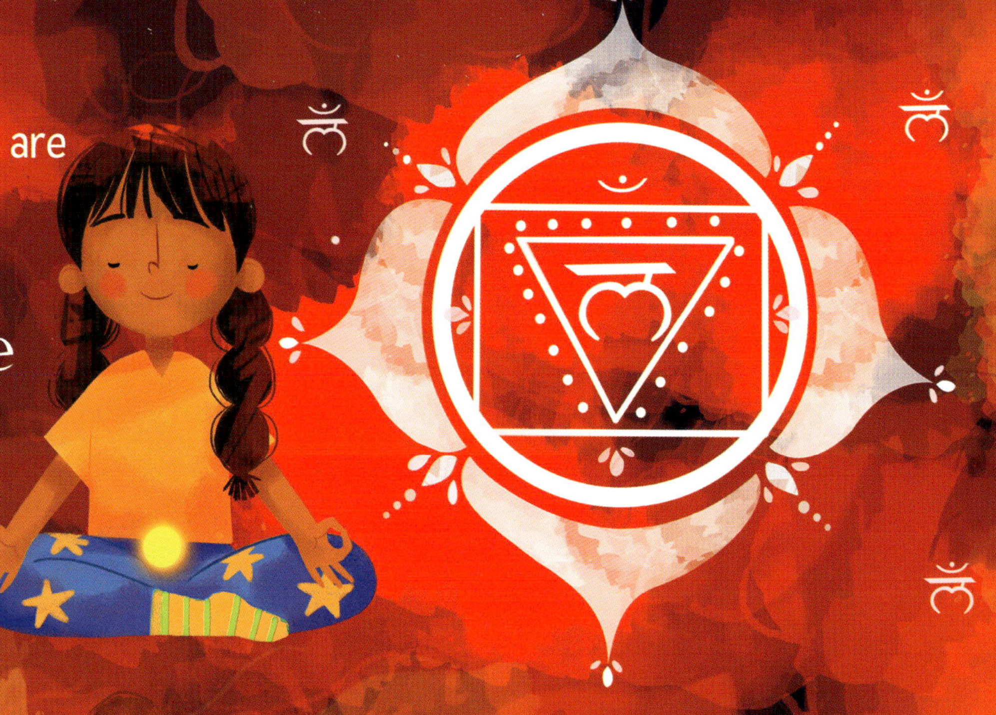

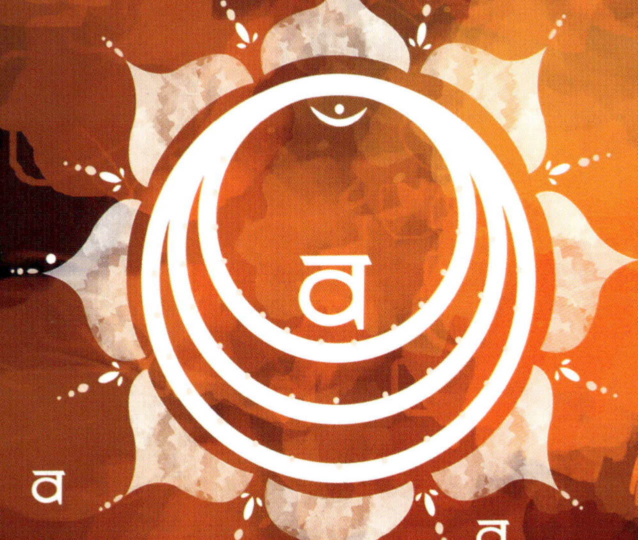

"The second chakra is under your bellybutton. This chakra balances your feelings."
"I feel excited to learn more about yoga" says Sam.

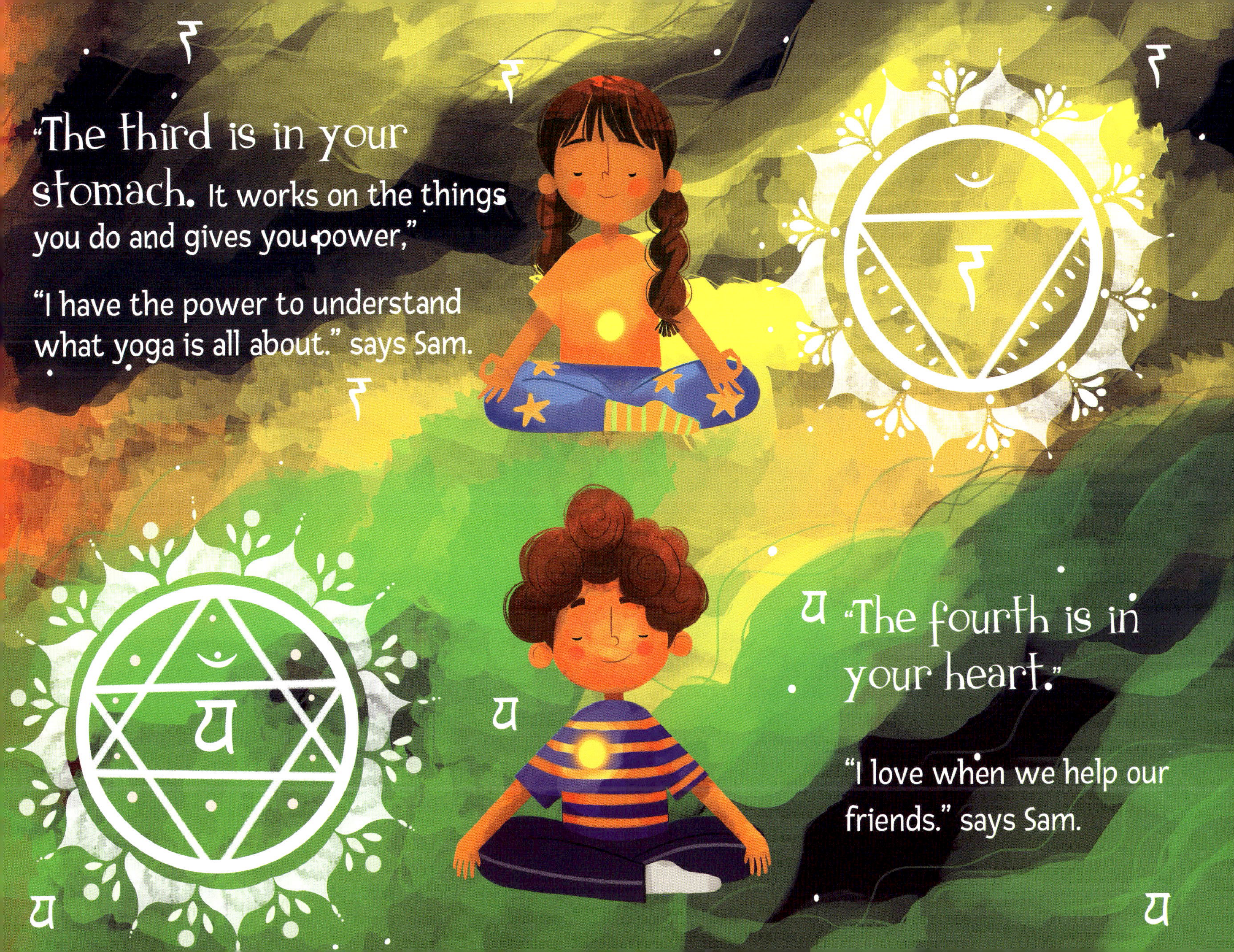

"The third is in your stomach. It works on the things you do and gives you power,"

"I have the power to understand what yoga is all about." says Sam.

"The fourth is in your heart."

"I love when we help our friends." says Sam.

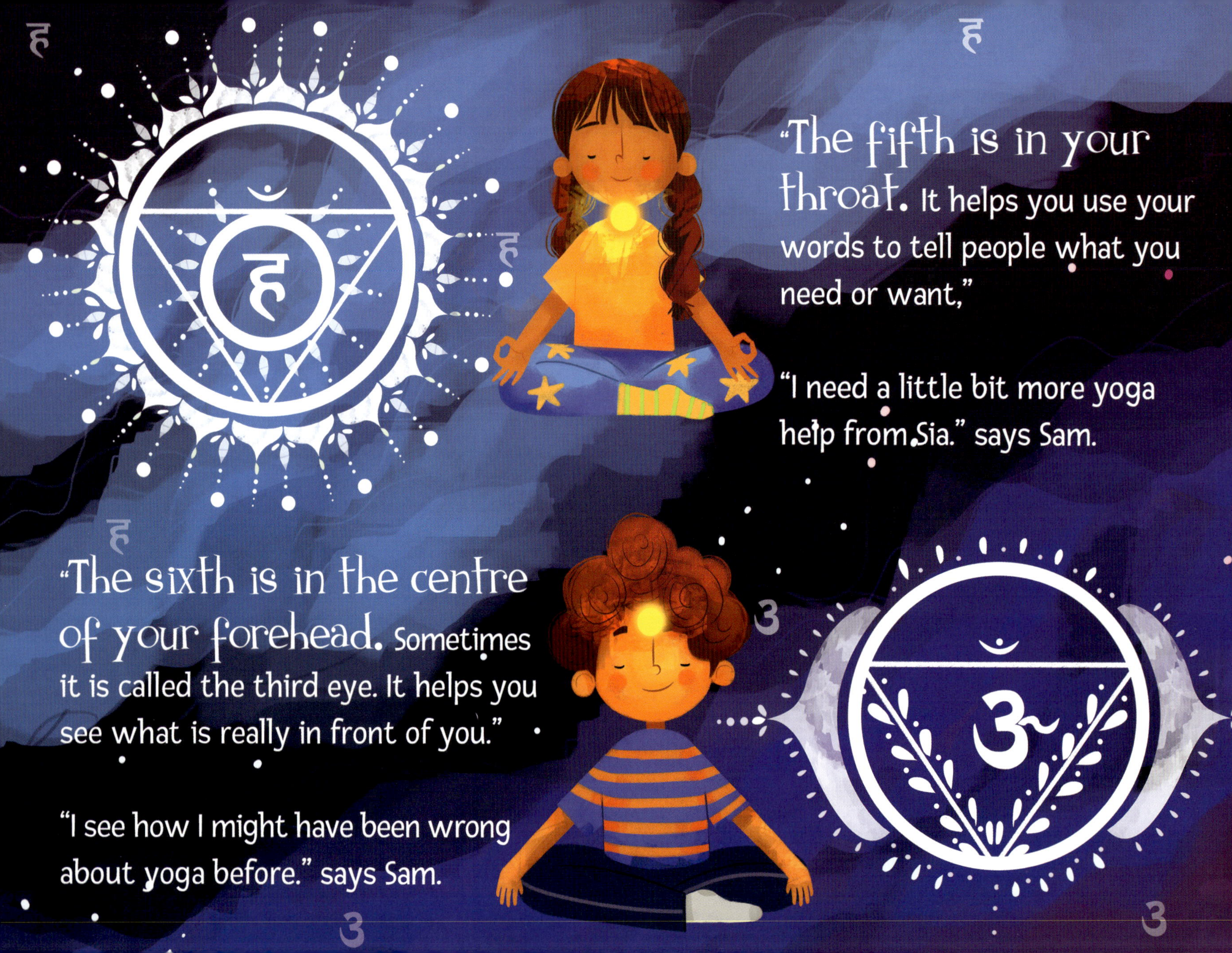

"The fifth is in your throat. It helps you use your words to tell people what you need or want,"

"I need a little bit more yoga help from Sia." says Sam.

"The sixth is in the centre of your forehead. Sometimes it is called the third eye. It helps you see what is really in front of you."

"I see how I might have been wrong about yoga before." says Sam.

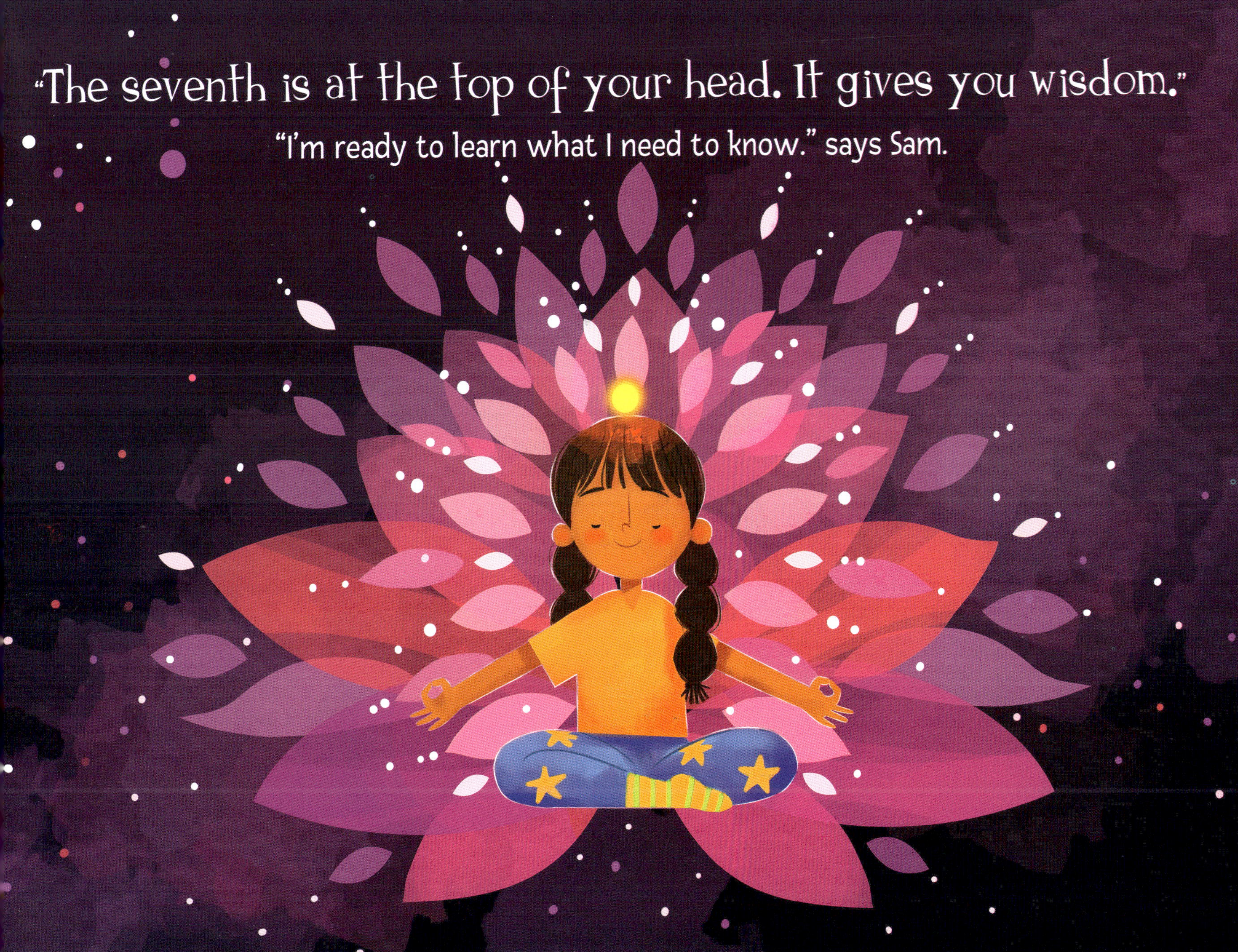

"The seventh is at the top of your head. It gives you wisdom."
"I'm ready to learn what I need to know." says Sam.

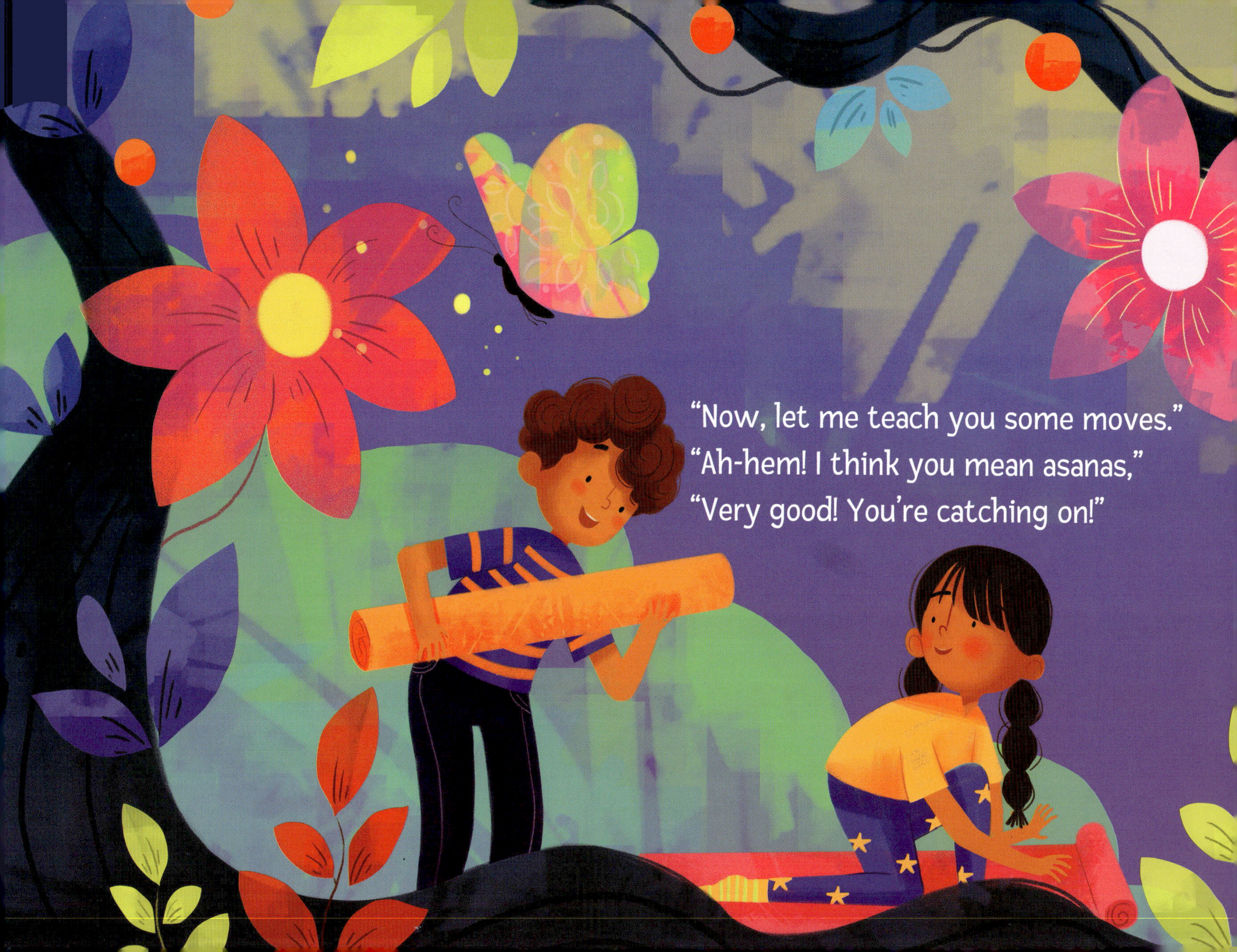

"Now, let me teach you some moves."
"Ah-hem! I think you mean asanas,"
"Very good! You're catching on!"

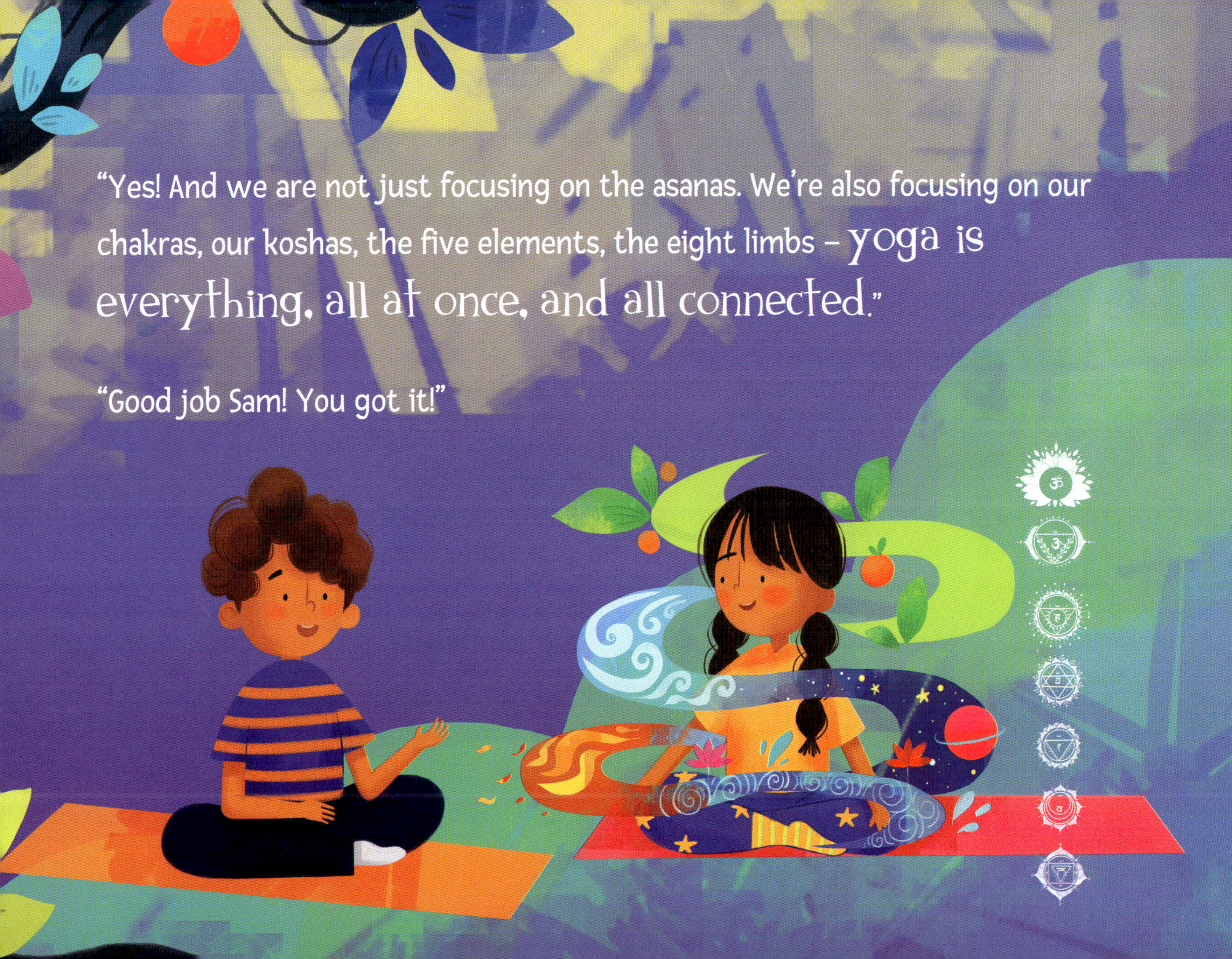

"Yes! And we are not just focusing on the asanas. We're also focusing on our chakras, our koshas, the five elements, the eight limbs – yoga is everything, all at once, and all connected."

"Good job Sam! You got it!"

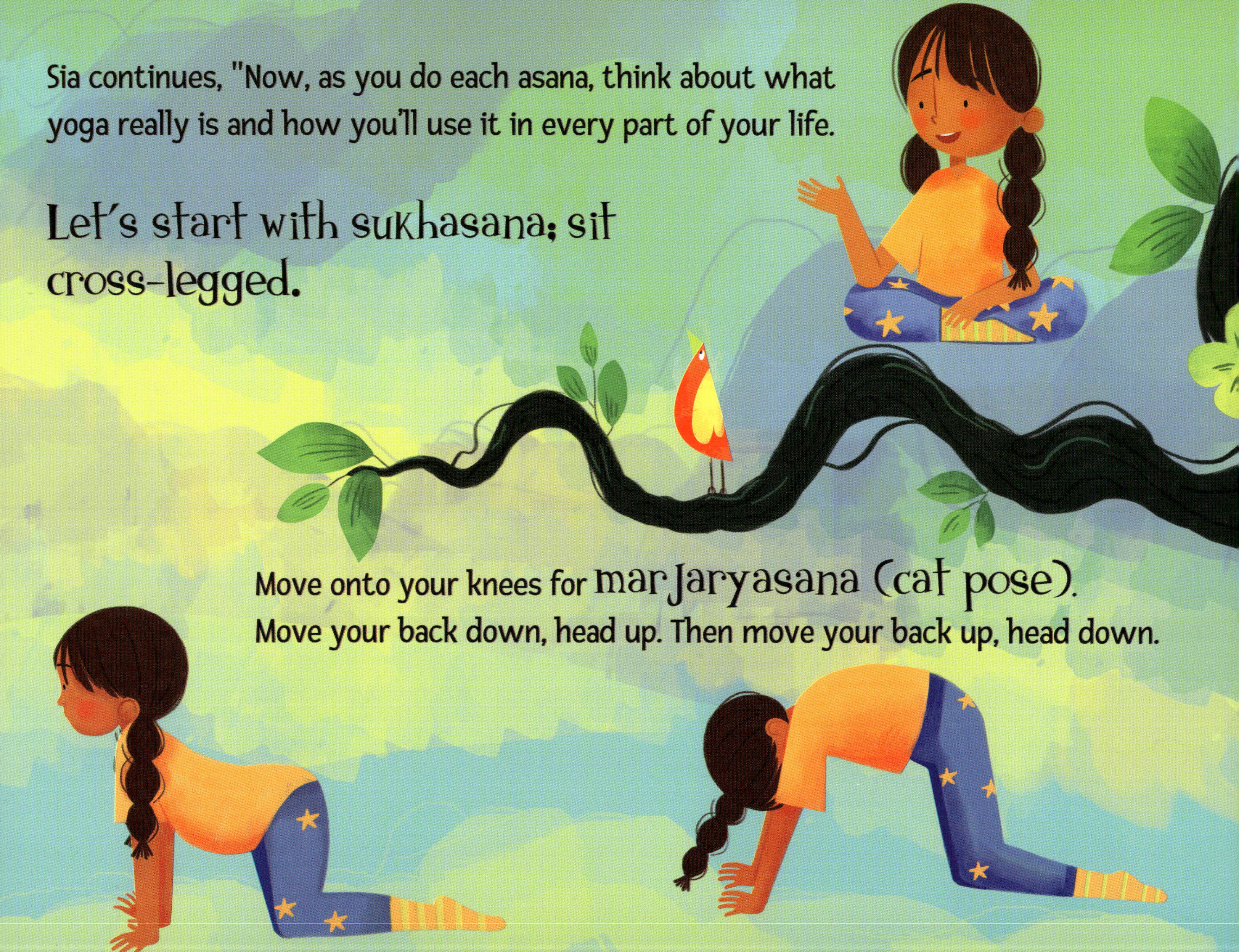

Sia continues, "Now, as you do each asana, think about what yoga really is and how you'll use it in every part of your life.

Let's start with sukhasana; sit cross-legged.

Move onto your knees for marjaryasana (cat pose). Move your back down, head up. Then move your back up, head down.

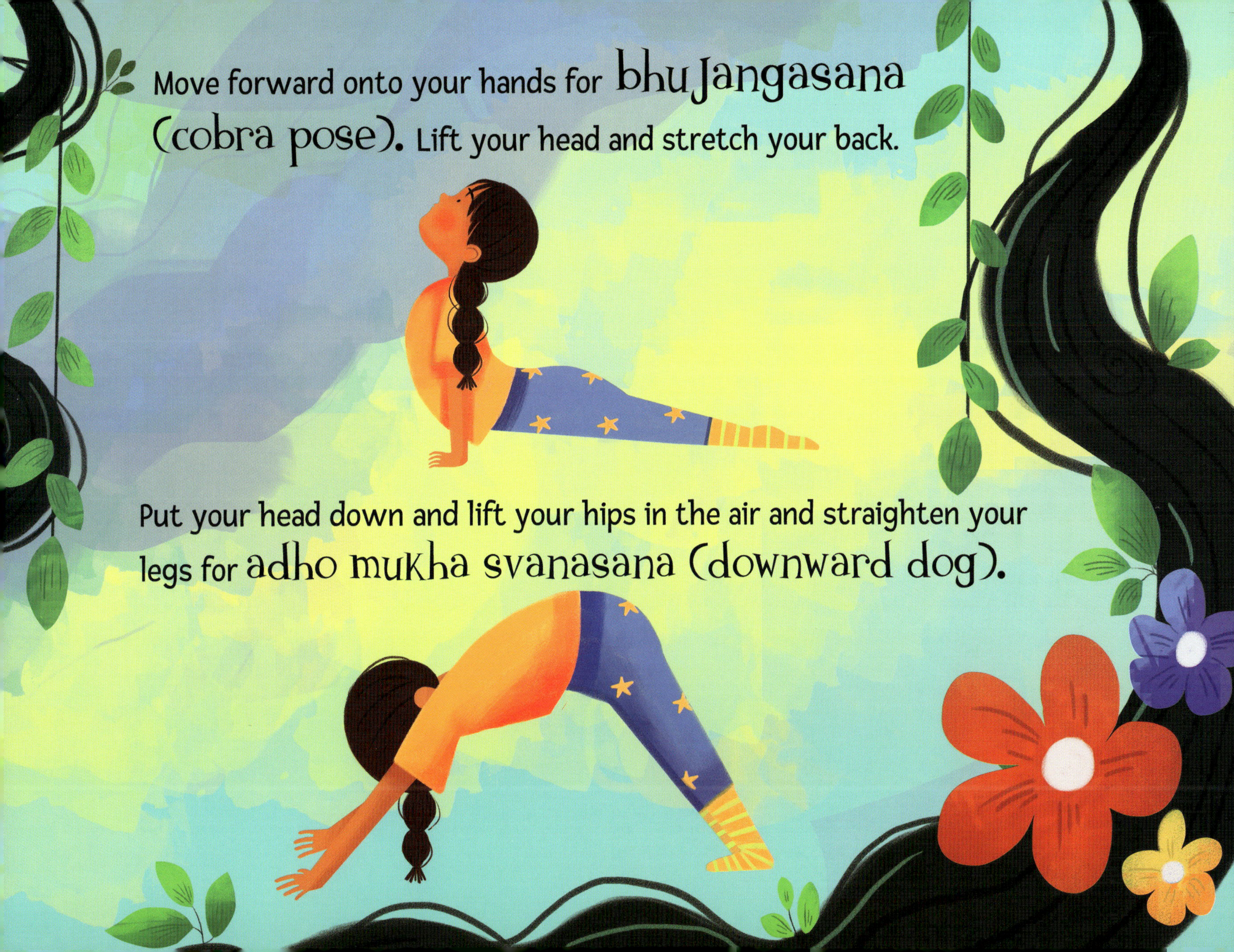

Move forward onto your hands for bhuJangasana (cobra pose). Lift your head and stretch your back.

Put your head down and lift your hips in the air and straighten your legs for adho mukha svanasana (downward dog).

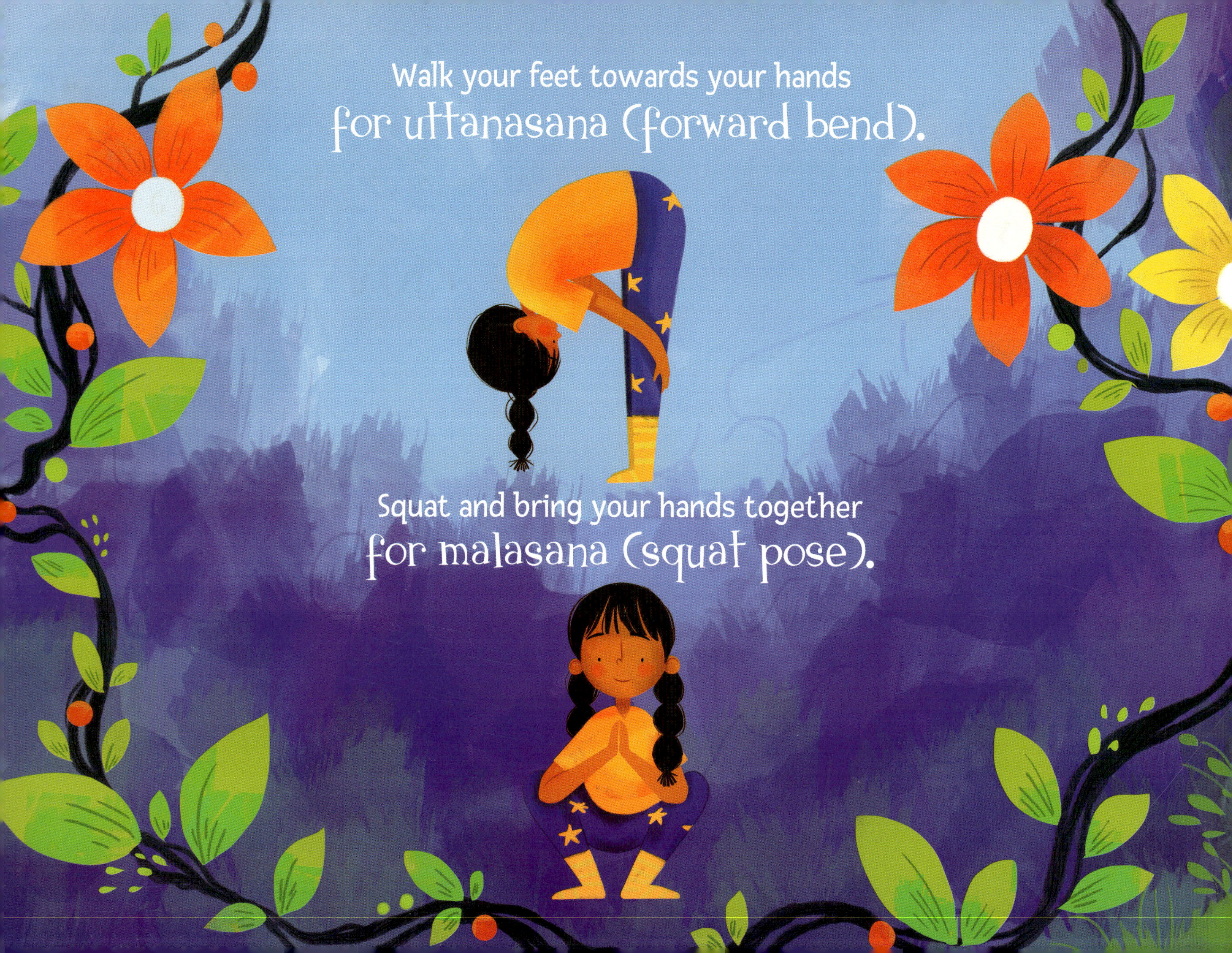

Walk your feet towards your hands
for uttanasana (forward bend).

Squat and bring your hands together
for malasana (squat pose).

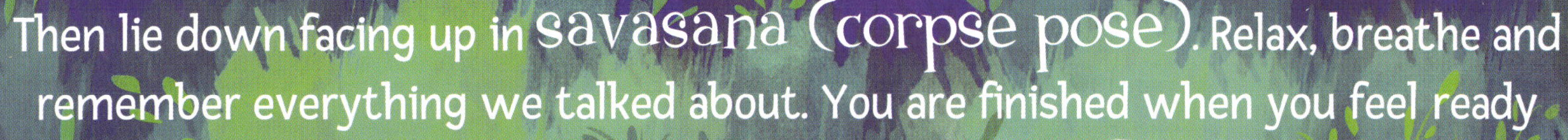

Then lie down facing up in savasana (corpse pose). Relax, breathe and remember everything we talked about. You are finished when you feel ready to get back up."

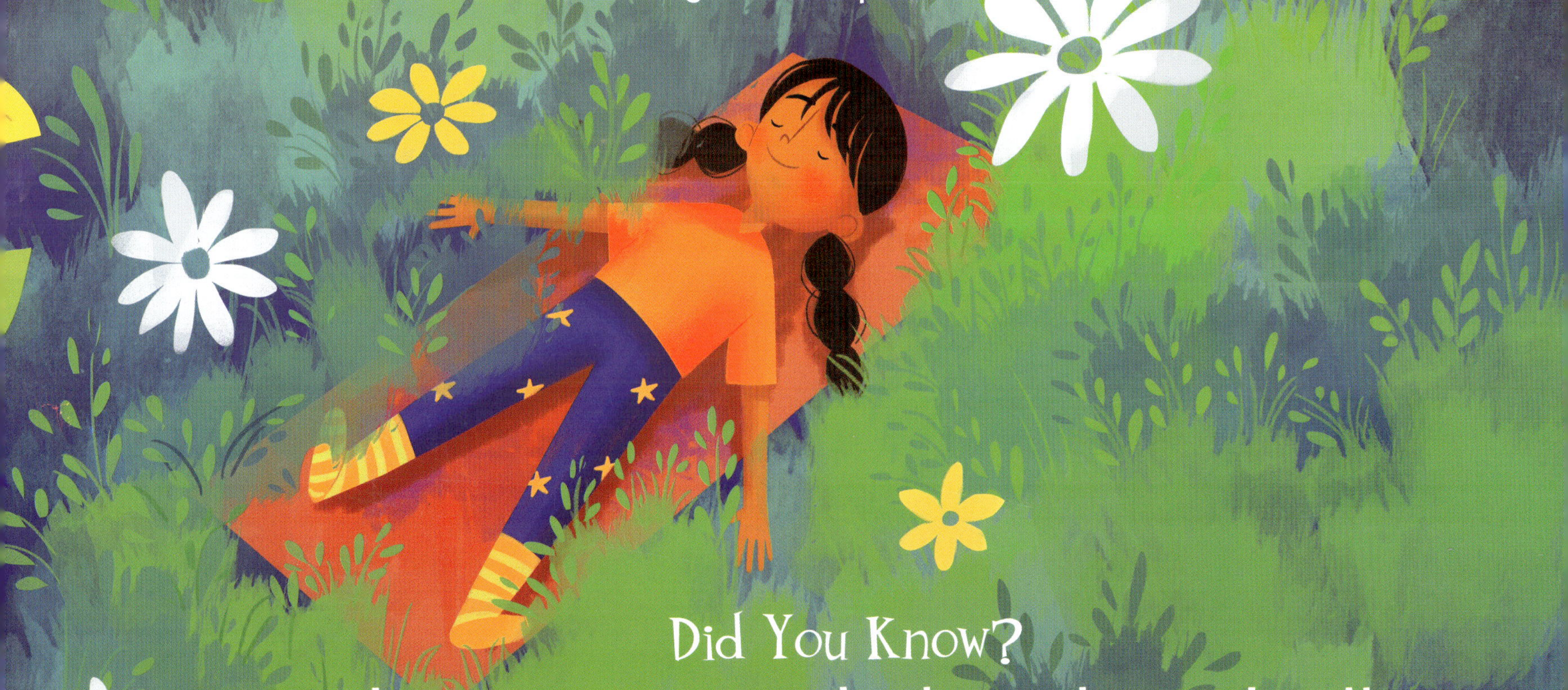

Did You Know?

Yoga Nidra is a yoga practice somewhere between being awake and being asleep. However, your mind is completely focused on what's going on in your body. Many yogis start in savasana, relax their bodies, minds, senses and emotions, and then enter yoga nidra.

Salutations, to the lineage of great Guru's.

Follow the authors on Instagram.